DASH DIET

Cookbook for beginners

Discover Delicious & Nutrient-Packed Recipes: A Beginner's Guide to the Dash Diet for Weight Loss and Heart Health

bristol poole

Contents

Introduction

Welcome to the Dash Diet World, where health meets flavor, and every meal is a celebration of well-being! In these pages, you'll embark on a culinary journey designed to nourish your body, delight your taste buds, and transform the way you approach food. The Dash Diet, short for Dietary Approaches to Stop Hypertension, isn't just about reducing sodium; it's a holistic approach to eating that emphasizes whole, nutrient-dense foods.

As you embark on this culinary adventure, you'll discover a treasure trove of delicious recipes carefully crafted to align with Dash Diet principles. Whether you're a seasoned pro at healthy living or just beginning to explore the world of balanced nutrition, this cookbook is your companion to making nutritious and mouthwatering meals a part of your daily routine.

About the Dash Diet

The Dash Diet has gained recognition for its effectiveness in promoting heart health and overall well-being. Originating as a dietary plan to manage hypertension, it has evolved into a comprehensive lifestyle approach. By focusing on an abundance of fruits, vegetables, lean proteins, and whole grains, the Dash Diet provides a roadmap to a balanced and heart-healthy way of eating.

What to Expect

In the following pages, you'll find a diverse array of recipes thoughtfully categorized to suit various tastes, preferences, and dietary needs. From energizing breakfasts to savory dinners, wholesome lunches to guilt-free snacks, and delightful desserts, each recipe is crafted with your health in mind without compromising on flavor.

How to Use This Cookbook

Navigating through this cookbook is designed to be effortless. Each recipe comes with clear instructions, ingredient lists, and nutritional information, making it easy for you to make informed choices. Whether you're a busy professional, a parent juggling multiple responsibilities, or someone with specific dietary preferences, there's a Dash Diet recipe here for you.

Enhancing Your Dash Diet Journey

To further support your Dash Diet journey, we've included informative sections on the fundamentals of the Dash Diet, practical tips for success, and even special occasion menus that allow you to celebrate while staying committed to your health goals.

Get ready to savor the benefits of a heart-healthy lifestyle. This cookbook is your passport to a world where nutritious choices meet culinary delight. Let's embark on this flavorful and wholesome journey together!

This cookbook is your companion on the path to adopting and savoring the Dash Diet. Whether you're a beginner exploring the fundamentals or a seasoned enthusiast seeking fresh inspiration, you'll find a diverse collection of recipes that cater to various tastes, preferences, and occasions.

Before you dive into the delicious world of Dash Diet recipes, take a moment to familiarize yourself with the essential guidelines, meal planning strategies, and kitchen tools that will make your culinary experience seamless and enjoyable. Discover the joy of preparing balanced, flavorful meals that not only contribute to your health but also bring joy to the table.

Get ready to explore breakfasts that energize your mornings, lunches that delight your taste buds, dinners that satisfy your cravings, and desserts that provide a sweet ending in moderation.

Whether you're hosting a gathering, planning for a special occasion, or simply enjoying a quiet meal at home, the Dash Diet principles will guide you towards making nutritious choices without compromising on flavor.

Let the journey begin, and may your Dash Diet adventure be a delectable and healthful exploration of the incredible world of wholesome eating!

Greetings from Dash Diet World

Overview

Welcome to the Dash Diet, a life-changing path that will help you become a healthier, more energetic version of yourself. We welcome you to embark on a culinary adventure where you will discover a world where health and deliciousness coexist side by side. Dietary Approaches to Stop Hypertension, or the Dash Diet, is more than simply a diet; it's a path to a healthy, balanced life.

An Overview of the Dash Diet

Beginnings and Development

The Dash Diet was born out of a dedication to health and a great deal of research on the management of hypertension. It has developed into a comprehensive way of living over time, recognising the connection between mindful eating and general health. This is a holistic approach to body and spirit nourishment, not just a diet.

Essential Ideas for the Dash Diet

The Dash Diet is based on the ideas of moderation and balance. The Dash Diet provides a path to a healthy lifestyle by emphasising nutrient-dense foods and reducing sodium consumption. It promotes a fulfilling and sustainable way of living, going beyond traditional ideas of dieting.

The Science of Nutrition in Dash
Blood Pressure Association

The Dash Diet's significant reduction in blood pressure is one of its main features. Focusing on the proper ratio of nutrients—in particular, potassium, magnesium, and calcium—makes the diet an effective tool for preserving normal blood pressure levels. Consequently, enhanced cardiovascular health and general energy are enhanced.

Heart-Rescuing Ingredients

The goal of the Dash Diet is to improve your cardiovascular health overall, not merely reduce your sodium intake. Including fruits, vegetables, whole grains, lean meats, and low-fat dairy not only strengthens the heart but also provides nourishment for the entire body. You're actively promoting wellbeing from the inside out, not just staving off illness

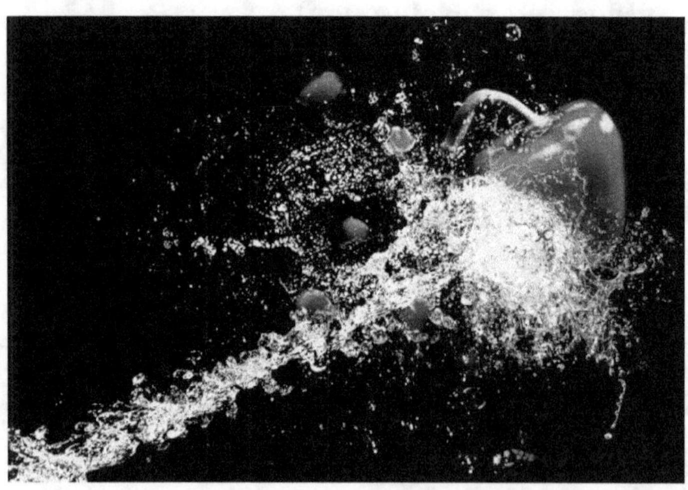

Introduction to Dash Guidelines

Sodium Consumption per Day

Understanding and following the salt guidelines of the Dash Diet gives you the power to take charge of your health. Reducing sodium consumption is more than just a dietary adjustment; it's a proactive move that can help lower blood pressure, support renal health, and enhance general vigour.

Recognizing Serving Sizes

A balanced diet that encourages the right portion amounts for every food category is the goal of the Dash Diet. This is about rethinking portion norms and creating a healthier relationship with food, not about imposing restrictive measures.

When you adopt the Dash Diet, you set out on a path that goes beyond the plate. It's about living a way that puts your health first, bringing life into every part of yourself. A world where every meal is an occasion to celebrate your health and every decision you make moves you closer to becoming a happier, healthier version of yourself

Learning About the Dash Guidelines

Recognizing Serving Sizes

An essential component of sticking to the Dash Diet is controlling your portion sizes, which guarantees that you'll keep a balanced and tasty diet. The following useful advice on portion management will improve your Dash Diet experience:

1. **Employ Visual Cues:** Acquaint yourself with visual signals so that you can gauge serving sizes. A cup of vegetables should be around the size of your fist, a portion of meat should be about

the size of a deck of cards, and a teaspoon of oil should be about the size of your thumb tip.

2. Calculate and Weigh: Get a kitchen scale, measuring cups, and spoons. Measuring *ingredients* precisely might make you more conscious of serving amounts, particularly when preparing meals at home.

3. Partitioning plates: Assign half of your plate to veggies, 25% to lean proteins, and the remaining 25% to whole grains or carbohydrates. This division should be made mentally. This easy rule guarantees a filling and well-balanced dinner.

4. Never Miss a Meal: Eating balanced, regular meals throughout the day can help reduce the risk of overindulging in later meals. Missing meals can cause extreme hunger, which makes portion control more difficult.

5. Pay Attention to Liquid Calories: When consuming beverages, especially those high in calories, be mindful of portion sizes. Reduce your intake of sugary drinks and choose low-calorie alternatives like water, herbal teas, or other beverages.

6. Prior to Portion Snacks: Portion snacks ahead of time into smaller containers or baggies rather than eating them straight out of the package. This helps regulate calorie intake and stops mindless eating.

7. Observe Your Hunger Cues: Eat mindfully, taking note of your body's signals of hunger and fullness. Not when the platter is empty, but rather when you are satisfied, stop eating. Your body needs some time to realize that it is full.

8. Keep an Eye Out for Hidden Calories: Watch out for toppings and condiments that are rich in calories. They can add extra calories even though they can improve flavor. Use them in moderation or choose more healthful options.

9. Select Tiny Plates: By making the plate appear fuller, using smaller plates can help regulate portion sizes and stop overeating.

10. Make a Plan: Arrange your snacks and meals ahead of time. It might help you avoid making rash decisions and maintain proper portion sizes to plan what and when you eat.

You can manage the Dash Diet rules more easily if you incorporate these portion control suggestions into your everyday routine. Recall that cultivating a sustainable and thoughtful eating habit is more important for long-term health and wellbeing than restricting oneself.

Managing Your Weight with the Dash Diet

Originally intended to treat hypertension, the Dash Diet has developed into a comprehensive lifestyle plan with significant weight-management implications. The Dash Diet helps with weight loss as well as weight maintenance in the following ways:

1. Stressing the Value of Nutrient-Dense Foods

• Nutrient-dense foods including fruits, vegetables, lean proteins, and entire grains are highlighted in the Dash Diet. These foods are perfect for managing weight since they are not only high in vital vitamins and minerals but also have a reduced calorie density.

2. Proper Macronutrient Balance:

• The diet promotes a macronutrient distribution that is balanced, with an emphasis on moderate intakes of complex crabs, lean proteins, and healthy fats. This equilibrium facilitates fullness and aids in avoiding overindulgence in any particular nutrient.

3. Principles of Portion Control:

• Recommendations for portion control are part of the Dash Diet, which is essential for successful weight management. Through comprehension of suitable serving sizes and implementation of portion control techniques, people can prevent consuming an excessive amount of calories.

4. Limitation on Foods Processed:

The Dash Diet forbids the eating of foods heavy in salt and processed. Processed foods can cause weight gain because they frequently include harmful fats and added sugars. Consuming complete, unadulterated foods helps people better regulate how many calories they consume.

5. Reduction of Sodium and Fluid Equilibrium:

• Although the Dash Diet is most known for its ability to control blood pressure, its concentration on cutting sodium intake also helps with weight management. Water retention can be caused by sodium, so lowering it may cause people to lose less water weight.

6. Encouragement of an Eco-Friendly Way of Life:

• The Dash Diet is a long-term way of living rather than a magic bullet. It promotes sustained adherence to a healthy diet, increasing the likelihood that people will keep the weight off in the long run.

7. Part of Heart-Healthy Exercise:

• A vital part of the Dash Diet's all-encompassing strategy, regular physical activity is not just a weight loss aid. By regulating calorie expenditure and promoting weight loss, exercise improves general health and facilitates weight maintenance.

8. Adaptable Method:

• The Dash Diet may be customized to fit each person's needs and tastes. The diet is flexible enough to accommodate a range of goals, whether the person is trying to lose weight, maintain a healthy weight, or just feel better overall.

By following the Dash Diet, people can efficiently control their weight while simultaneously developing a lifestyle that supports long-term health and vitality. The diet is a viable option for anyone looking for weight management strategies since it promotes a balanced and thoughtful relationship with food rather than harsh limits.

Rewards for Wellness and Health
Achievements and Practical Instances

Observing the Dash Diet's life-changing effects on people offers strong proof of its effectiveness. The following success stories highlight the real advantages of leading a heart-healthy lifestyle:

1. The Path to Lower Blood Pressure:

• Meet Sarah, whose blood pressure significantly decreased after adhering to the Dash Diet consistently. Her success story serves as evidence of the strong link between cardiovascular health and food decisions.

2. Heart Health and Loss of Weight:

John's experience serves as an example of how the Dash Diet promotes cardiac heath in addition to weight loss. He lost weight by embracing heart-healthy eating practices, and he also saw improvements in his cholesterol and general cardiovascular health.

3. Taking Care of Heart Health with Diabetes:

• Maria, who was given a diabetes diagnosis, learned that following the Dash Diet would help her priorities heart health and control her blood sugar levels. Her experience highlights how adaptable the diet is in treating a range of health issues.

4. Benefits for the entire family:

• The Anderson family's dedication to following the Dash Diet resulted in a group effort to improve heart health. Their combined experiences demonstrate how putting the diet's ideas into practice may have a positive effect on the health of an entire family.

Advantages of Cardiovascular
The Science of Nutrition in Dash

Blood Pressure Association

The primary way that the Dash Diet affects heart health is by controlling blood pressure:

1. Lowering Sodium to Manage Blood Pressure:

• The diet's focus on cutting back on sodium consumption is essential for preserving normal blood pressure levels. Adhering to the Dash Diet principles is positively correlated with blood pressure management, as demonstrated by several real-world cases.

2. Phosphorous, Magnesium- and Calcium-Rich:

• Dietary items that follow the Dash Diet are naturally high in calcium, magnesium, and potassium—minerals that are vital for heart health. Examples from everyday life show how these nutrients support better heart health and a lower risk of heart disease.

Heart-Rescuing Ingredients

.A Comprehensive Strategy for Heart Health:

• Read about the experiences of people whose heart wellness has improved overall by implementing the Dash Diet principles. In addition to controlling blood pressure, these people have shown improvements in triglycerides, cholesterol, and heart health in general.

Stress the Long-Term Advantages:

1. Transformation of a Sustainable Lifestyle

• Pay attention to people who have made the Dash Diet their permanent way of life. Their experiences demonstrate the long-term cardiovascular benefits of maintaining heart-healthy practices, supporting the notion that the Dash Diet is a long-term rather than a short-term treatment.

2. Decreased Chance of Cardiovascular Conditions:

• Showcase empirical evidence and statistical data illustrating how long-term adherence to the Dash Diet can dramatically lower the risk of cardiovascular illnesses. Stress that investing in heart health will pay off by granting you a longer, healthier life.

The Dash Diet's nutritional science is combined with real-world success stories to help readers visualize the immediate and long-term advantages of leading this heart-healthy lifestyle.

How to Use the Cookbook
Classification of Recipes

Take a gastronomic trip with our well arranged cookbook, which is meant to make your Dash Diet experience easier. For your convenience, we have organized the recipes as follows:

1. Categories of Meals:

• *Breakfast Bliss*: Start your days off well with nutritious breakfast selections.

• *Lunch Delights*: Try out a selection of savoury and fresh lunch meals.

• *Dinner Wonders*: Treat yourself to a filling and healthy dinner to cap offs your day.

• *Snacks and Sides*: Enjoy tasty side dishes and wholesome snacks for any occasion.

• *Desserts for Dash Enthusiasts*: Treat your sweet tooth to something guilt-free.

2. Menus for Special Occasions:

• *Holiday Feasts:* Use Dash Diet-approved holiday recipes to provide a festive touch to your get-togethers.

• *Festive Occasions:* Mark important days with recipes designed to keep you on the heart-healthy celebration road.

3. Nutritional Limitations:

• *Vegetarian Options:* Discover delicious plant-based foods that are appropriate for vegans and vegetarians.

• *Gluten-Free Goodness:* Savour meals that are free of gluten and suitable for a variety of diets.

• *Low-Sodium Creations:* Savour tasty dishes made with low sodium content for individuals who priorities low sodium diets.

It's simple to locate recipes that meet your individual requirements because each category has been carefully designed to accommodate your dietary choices.

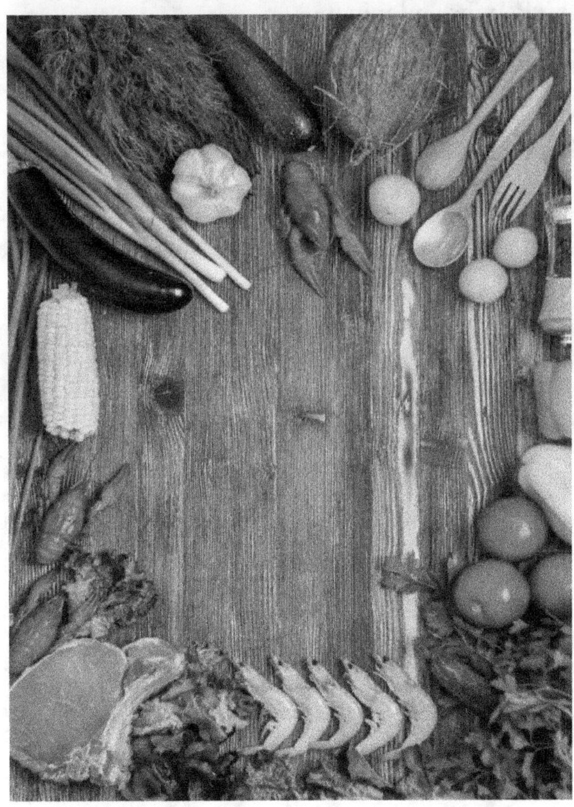

Getting Around the Recipe Book
Ingredient Vocabulary

Use our extensive Ingredient Glossary to uncover the mysteries behind the recipes created with the Dash Diet. Here, we explore the essential elements that combine to create each recipe's exquisite flavour and wealth of nutritious benefits:

1. Produce and Fruits:

• *Berries:* Packed with fibre and antioxidants, berries liven up your food and offer several health advantages.

• *Leafy Greens:* The foundation of a healthy diet, these greens are bursting with vitamins and minerals.

2. Proteins:

• *Lean Poultry:* Rich in protein but low in fat, this food type supports healthy muscles.

• *Legumes:* Packed with protein and fibre, legumes support general wellbeing and satiety.

3. Complete Grains:

• *Quinoa:* A multipurpose grain rich in critical amino acids and protein.

• *Brown rice:* A heart-healthy, high-fiber substitute for refined grains.

4. Dairy and Substitutes:

• *Greek Yoghurt:* This high-calcium choice gives your meals creaminess and probiotics.

• **_Almond milk:_** A dairy-free substitute that has extra minerals and vitamins.

5. Spices and Herbs:

• **_Turmeric:_** Added to food, turmeric has anti-inflammatory qualities and gives it depth and colour.

• **_Garlic:_** Known for its possible cardiovascular benefits, garlic is not merely a flavour enhancer.

6. Good Fat s:

• **_Avocado_**: A heart-healthy, nutrient-dense source of monounsaturated fats.

• **_Olive oil:_** Rich in healthy fats and antioxidants, it improves flavour and overall wellbeing.

We give you comprehensive information on the nutritional advantages of each ingredient so you can make wise decisions when preparing delicious, heart-healthy meals. As you prepare meals that satiate your body and spirit, let the Ingredient Glossary be your guide

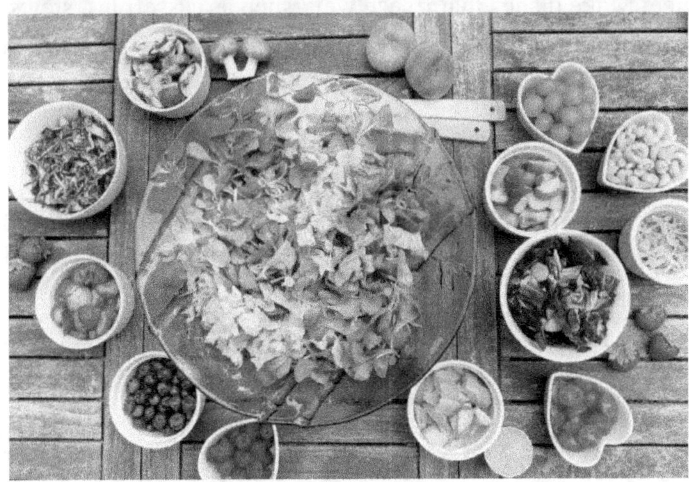

Useful Advice and Meal Scheduling

Strategies for Meal Preparation

Our time-saving meal prep techniques combine efficiency and nutrition to create a seamless Dash Diet regimen that fits into your daily routine:

1. Weekly Scheduling:

• *Pro Tip*: Set aside a particular day of the week for grocery shopping and meal preparation. A well-thought-out plan helps you make fewer decisions during the workweek.

2. Cooking in batches:

• Pro tip: Make big batches of basic items like roasted veggies, lean meats, and nutritious grains. Keep them divided into portions so you can quickly put them together on hectic days.

3. Low-Freezer Dinners:

• Advice: Make dishes that freeze well, such as casseroles, stews, and soups. These are quite easy to reheat, which saves time when making meals from scratch is difficult.

4. Ready-Cut Vegetables:

• Pro tip: Prepare veggies ahead of time by cutting and storing them. This makes dinner preparation easier and guarantees that you always have a rainbow of vibrant vegetables on hand.

5. Employ Instant Pots and Slow Cookers:

• **Pro Tip:** Delegate the task to your Instant Pot or slow cooker. Prepare it in the morning and come home to a flavorful, prepared meal.

Keeping Nutrients Balanced at Every Meal

The main goal of the Dash Diet is to achieve a balanced, nutrient-rich diet. For best health, balance your macronutrients as follows:

1. Include Vibrant Vegetables:

• *Tip:* Try to include a variety of vibrant vegetables on half of your plate. They improve general health since they are high in fibre, vitamins, and minerals.

2. Trim Proteins:

• Advice: Make sure your meals contain lean protein sources including fish, chicken, beans, and lentils. Protein keeps you feeling full and helps maintain the health of your muscles.

3. Complete Grains:

• *Pro tip:* For complex carbohydrates, fibre, and important nutrients, goes for whole grains like brown rice, quinoa, and whole wheat bread.

4. Good Fats:

• *Tip:* To promote heart health and improve the flavour of your dishes, include sources of healthy fats in your diet, such as avocados, almonds, and olive oil.

5. Control of Portion:

• *Advice:* Pay attention to portion proportions to prevent overindulging. Utilise smaller plates and pay attention to your body's signals of fullness and hunger.

6. Healthy Snacks:

• *Advice*: Make sure your snacks are well-balanced, with a mix of fibre, protein, and good fats. In between meals, this helps sustain energy levels.

7. Drinking plenty of water

• *Advice:* Remember to stay hydrated. Water can help you feel full and is necessary for good health in general.

8. Turn Around Your Protein Sources:

• *Advice*: To guarantee a varied spectrum of nutrients, rotate your protein sources over the course of the week. This makes your meals more interesting as well.

You may make following the Dash Diet easier and improve the nutritional value of your meals while also improving your general health by putting these helpful suggestions into practice and concentrating on nutrient balance.

Essentials of the Dash Diet

The Dash Diet: *What Is It?*

Set out on a quest to learn the fundamentals of the Dash Diet and how it can drastically improve your health.

Overview of the Dash Diet

• **Meaning and Origin:** Dietary Approaches to Stop Hypertension, or the Dash Diet, was created as a means of lowering high blood pressure. Discover the history of this eating strategy and its scientific underpinnings.

Evolution of Focus: Follow the development of the Dash Diet from a focused strategy for hypertension management to an all-encompassing way of living. Recognise how its original intent has been expanded to encompass greater health and well-being.

Important Elements: Discover the underlying ideas that make the Dash Diet a nutrition and health trailblazer.

The Focus Is on Foods High in Nutrients:

• **Fruits & Vegetables:** Explore the cornerstone of the Dash Diet, which emphasises fruits and vegetables heavily. Find out how their abundance of vitamins, minerals, and antioxidants support general health.

• **Lean Proteins:** Recognise how important it is to include lean proteins in your diet, such as fish, chicken, beans, and lentils. Examine how protein affects satiety and muscular health.

• **Whole Grains:** Benefit from the high fibre content and long-lasting energy of whole grains like quinoa and brown rice. Find out how they promote heart health.

• **Dairy and Substitutes:** To ensure a balanced intake of vital nutrients, consider incorporating low-fat dairy products and substitutes.

• **Fruit and Vegetable Guidelines:** Learn about the suggested daily allowances of fruits and vegetables. Find inventive ways to add these essential *ingredients* to every meal.

• **Balancing Lean Proteins:** Find out how much lean protein is best served to satisfy your needs nutritionally and to support heart health.

• **Whole Grains for Sustenance:** Recognise the appropriate daily intake of whole grains to promote a healthy, well-balanced diet.

• **Moderation in Dairy:** Follow the recommendations for dairy and its substitutes to make sure your diet is well-rounded and heart-healthy.

Take hold of the guiding principles that will help you make decisions that will lead to a more lively and healthy living as you start your Dash Diet adventure. Accept the abundance of nutrients provided by nature's abundance and allow the Dash Diet to serve as your guide for long-term health.

The Science behind Dash: *How it works:*

Examine the Dash Diet's scientific foundations and discover how it affects health and wellbeing.

Controlling Blood Pressure

• ***Composition of Nutrients***: *Examine the ways in which the nutrient-dense Dash Diet—with its special focus on potassium, calcium, and magnesium—helps to regulate blood pressure.*

• *Recognize how these vital nutrients help the body's natural blood pressure-regulating systems and preserve artery health.*

• ***Potassium-Sodium Equilibrium:***

• *Get knowledge about the Dash Diet's crucial sodium-potassium balance. Learn how consuming more foods high in potassium and less salt promotes a balanced environment that is essential for cardiovascular health.*

• *Learn about the science underlying the interactions between these minerals and how they affect arterial flexibility, fluid balance, and the stability of blood pressure overall.*

Advantages for Cardiovascular Health

• **Heart Health in General:** Recognize that the Dash Diet offers several cardiovascular advantages beyond controlling blood pressure. Examine the ways in which a nutrient-dense diet might improve vascular health, triglyceride levels, and cholesterol.

• *Examine the defense mechanisms*, such as anti-inflammatory qualities and support for ideal vascular function that advance general heart health.

• **Lowering the Risk of Cardiovascular Disease:** Have a conversation about how following the Dash Diet can dramatically lower the risk of cardiovascular illnesses. Examine empirical research and case studies that demonstrate the association between long-term Dash Diet compliance and a lower risk of heart-related problems.

• *Take into account how nutrition might help reduce risk factors that lead to cardiovascular disease, such as inflammation, diabetes, and obesity.*

Introduction: Crucial Pointers

Arm yourself with the core principles need to begin a Dash Diet journey that works:

• **Sodium Intake per Day:** Recognize how crucial it is to control sodium intake for optimum health. Examine suggested daily allowances and workable methods to cut back on sodium in your meals.

• **Being Aware of Serving Sizes:** Recognize how important portion control is to the Dash Diet. Discover how adhering to the

Dash Diet's tenets and ensuring a balanced nutritional intake are achieved by understanding serving sizes.

• **Neutralizing Nutrients:** Master the art of preparing nutrient-dense, well-rounded meals. Learn how to balance macronutrients including fats, proteins, and crabs to promote general health.

• **Utensils and Substances**: Become familiar with the necessary supplies and components that makes sticking to the Dash Diet easier. Establish a kitchen atmosphere that promotes healthful food preparation and cooking.

With a firm grasp of the fundamental principles, practical tools, and scientific underpinnings required to promote a healthier and more heart-conscious lifestyle, you may confidently embark on your Dash Diet adventure.

Equipment and Substances

Learn about the vital components and tools that can support you on your Dash Diet path to a more aware and health-conscious way of living.

Sodium Consumption per Day

• **Suggested Sodium Limitations**: Recognizing the Threshold: Learn about the daily salt intake guidelines suggested by medical experts. Learn more about sodium's function in controlling blood pressure and its possible effects on cardiovascular health.

• **Adapting to Individual Needs:** Be aware that while recommendations for sodium intake are meant to serve as a general guideline for heart health, individual needs may differ.

Some Useful Advice for Lowering Sodium:

• **Herb and Spice Substitutes:** Discover a variety of tasty herbs and spices that can be used in place of salt. Find out how they can improve the flavor of your food without sacrificing your health.

• **Mindful Label Reading:** Learn how to recognize high-sodium foods by carefully reading food labels. Discover the hidden sources of salt in processed foods and shop with knowledge.

Recognizing Serving Sizes
Suggestions for Proper Serving Sizes

• **Balanced Meal Components:** Recognize the guidelines for serving sizes in each food group provided by the Dash Diet. Discover how to prepare meals that are well-balanced by using the appropriate amounts of nutritious grains, lean meats, fruits, and vegetables.

• **Visual clues:** Use visual clues to help you determine the right portion proportions. Allow straightforward illustrations to direct your meal planning, from protein portions to vegetable servings.

Portion Control Advice

• **Mindful Eating Practices:** Develop mindful eating techniques to improve your awareness of your body's signals of hunger and fullness. This stops overeating and encourages a better connection with food.

• **Use of Smaller Plates:** To naturally regulate portion amounts, use smaller plates. This psychological ploy promotes contentment with smaller portions.

Key Resources for People on Dash Diets:
Overview of Kitchen Appliances

• **Nutrient-Rich Food Preparation:** Learn about the necessary kitchen tools that make it easier to prepare meals that are high in nutrients. These appliances, which range from steamers for veggies to blenders for smoothies, make it easier to implement Dash Diet ideas.

• *Advice for Creating a Kitchen That's Dash Diet-Friendly:*

• **Organizational Strategies:** Get useful advice on how to arrange your kitchen in a way that adheres to the Dash Diet's tenets. Arrange your cutlery and pantry in a thoughtful manner to increase the accessibility and convenience of healthy options.

Ingredients for Dash Diet:
Summary of Essential Ingredients:

• **Staples for Healthier Living:** Examine a thorough rundown of essential components to have in your refrigerator and pantry. Learn how these staples—from lean proteins to nutritious grains—form the basis of a diet that promotes heart health.

• **Emphasis on Fresh and healthy Foods:** Stress the value of incorporating fresh and healthy foods into Dash Diet dishes. Find out how adding these components to your meals can improve their flavor while also improving your nutrition.

Set out on the Dash Diet with a comprehensive understanding of suggested sodium intake limits, advice on portion control, and insights into key components and tools. These useful components will enable you to make well-informed decisions and turn your kitchen into a centre of life and wellness.

Furnishing the Kitchen

Essential Kitchen Items for Those on a Dash: With these indispensable equipment, you can turn your kitchen into a centre of culinary creativity and health:

High-Grade Cookware

• **Non-Stick Pans:** Learn how using non-stick pans can help prepare meals in a healthy way. Examine how they facilitate simple cleanup and lessen the need for extra oil.

• **Steamer Baskets:** Use steamer baskets for a cooking technique that retains nutrients. Find out how steaming improves the tastes and textures of veggies and helps you maintain a balanced Dash Diet.

Advice for Selecting Kitchen Utensils:

• **Sturdy and Versatile:** Choose kitchen utensils that are both sturdy and adaptable with our advice. Invest in durable instruments that will assist your Dash Diet efforts, such as chopping boards and knives.

• **Boosting Nutrient-Packed meals:** Learn how to make your Dash Diet meals better with a food processor and blender. These tools improve kitchen efficiency by making nutrient-dense sauces and smoothies using fresh fruit.

• **Selecting the Correct Appliances:** Based on your cooking requirements, get advice on which food processor and blender to buy. Choose appliances that complement your culinary objectives, whether it's strong blending skills or accurate chopping.

Conscientious Food Buying

Use a Dash Diet mentality when navigating the aisles to make sure your food shopping advances your health objectives:

Making a shopping list for the Dash Diet

• **Meal preparing Advice:** Master the skill of organizing your grocery list by preparing meals in advance. Anticipate your needs for the entire week to streamline your food shopping experience.

The Significance of Following Your List: Stress how important it is to follow your shopping list. Remain committed to making healthy decisions by abstaining from impulsive purchases and adhering to your list of things.

Getting Around the Islands:

• **Choosing Fresh Produce:** Find out how to choose fresh produce that complies with the Dash Diet's tenets. Investigate the colorful world of fruits and vegetables, making sure that the foods you choose will contribute to a diet rich in color and nutrients.

• **Techniques for Making Healthier Decisions:** Create techniques for navigating the aisles that highlight the significance of choosing whole grains and lean proteins. Discover which processed and high-sodium foods to steer clear of in order to meet your Dash Diet objectives.

Advice for Meal Planning

Learn how to create a weekly menu that is balanced and varied to help you stick to the Dash Diet:

Weekly Meal Schedule:

• **Step-by-Step Guide:** To plan meals for the coming week, adhere to an extensive, step-by-step guide. Make sure every meal, from breakfast to supper, offers a balanced nutritional profile and complies with the Dash Diet's tenets.

• **Including Variety and Balance:** Make sure your weekly menu has both. Learn how to add a variety of food groups, hues, and textures to your meals to make them interesting and filling.

Cooking and Freezing in Bulk

• **Time-Saving Advice:** Take advantage of batch cooking's advantages to save time on hectic days. Discover time-saving techniques for cooking big meals that may be frozen for later use.

• **Preserving Quality through Freezing:** Learn how to freeze your Dash Diet meals properly to preserve their quality. Make sure frozen meals maintain their flavors and nutritional content for quick, wholesome dinners.

Prepare yourself with the information and resources necessary to organize your kitchen to fit the Dash Diet, shop for groceries purposefully, and become an expert meal planner for long-term success on your health journey.

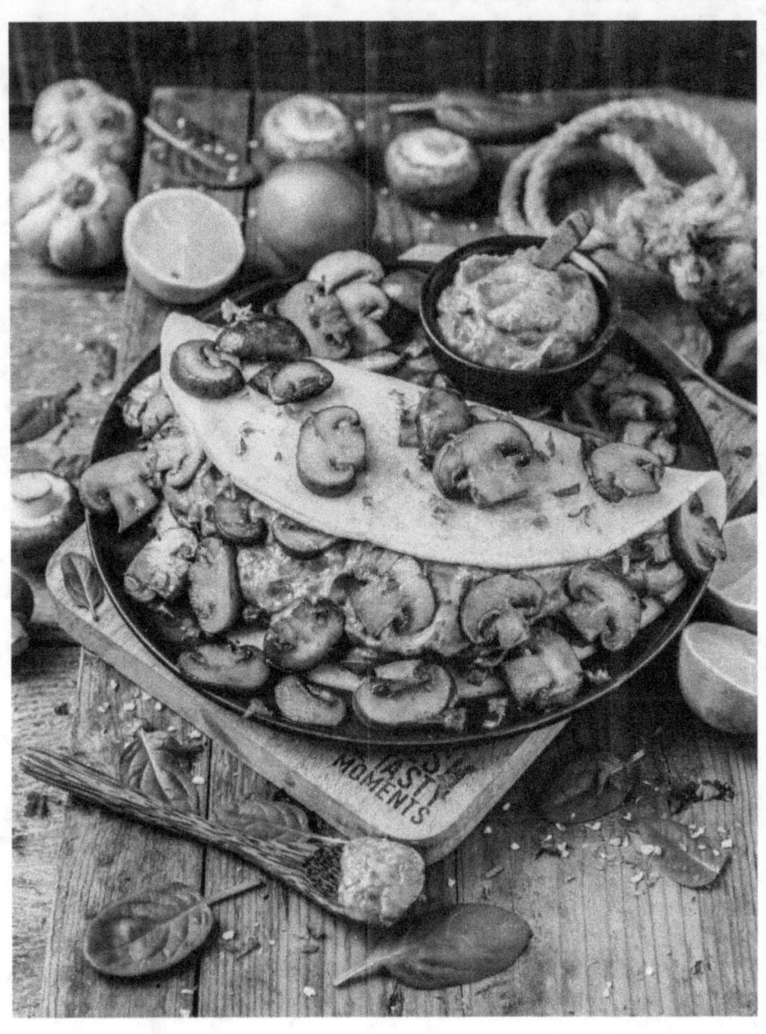

Breakfast Bliss

Quick and Easy Morning Oats

Preparation Time: 5 minutes
Cooking Time: 5 minutes
Yield: 1 serving

Ingredients:

- 1/2 cup rolled oats
- 1 cup unsweetened almond milk
- 1/2 cup fresh strawberries, sliced
- 2 tablespoons Greek yogurt
- 1 tablespoon chia seeds
- 1 teaspoon honey (optional)
- A sprinkle of cinnamon

Procedure:

1. **Prepare *Ingredients*:**
   - Gather all the ***ingredients*** and have them measured and ready for use.
2. **Cooking Oats:**
   - In a small saucepan, combine rolled oats and almond milk.
   - Bring the mixture to a gentle boil over medium heat, stirring occasionally.
3. **Simmer and Stir:**
   - Once boiling, reduce heat to low and simmer for about 3-5 minutes or until the oats reach your desired consistency.
   - Stir frequently to prevent sticking.
4. **Assemble the Bowl:**
   - Transfer the cooked oats to a serving bowl.
5. **Add Toppings:**
   - Top the oats with sliced strawberries, Greek yogurt, chia seeds, and a drizzle of honey if desired.
6. **Final Touch:**

- Sprinkle a dash of cinnamon over the top for added flavor.

7. **Serve and Enjoy:**
    - Your Quick and Easy Morning Oats are ready to be served! Enjoy a nutritious and delicious start to your day.

Tips and Variations:

- Customize with Your Favorite Fruits: Experiment with different fruits like blueberries, raspberries, or sliced banana.
- Adjust Sweetness: Tailor the sweetness to your liking by adjusting the amount of honey or opting for natural sweetness from fruits.
- Nutritional Boost: Add a tablespoon of nuts or seeds for an extra nutritional boost and crunch.
- Make-Ahead Option: Prepare a larger batch and refrigerate in individual jars for a quick grab-and-go breakfast during busy mornings.

Note: This recipe is designed to fit the Dash Diet principles with whole grains, low-fat dairy (Greek yogurt), and the incorporation of fresh fruits and seeds for added nutrients. Adjust portion sizes as needed for your dietary requirements.

Veggie-Packed Omelet

Preparation Time: 10 minutes
Cooking Time: 5 minutes
Yield: 1 serving

Ingredients:

- 2 large eggs
- 1/4 cup bell peppers, diced
- 1/4 cup cherry tomatoes, halved
- 1/4 cup spinach, chopped
- 2 tablespoons feta cheese, crumbled
- Salt and pepper to taste
- 1 teaspoon olive oil

Procedure:

1. **Prepare *Ingredients*:**
   - Dice bell peppers, halve cherry tomatoes, chop spinach, and crumble feta cheese.
2. **Preheat Pan:**
   - Heat olive oil in a non-stick skillet over medium heat.
3. **Saute Veggies:**
   - Add bell peppers to the pan and sauté for 2 minutes until slightly softened.
   - Add cherry tomatoes and spinach, sauté for an additional 1-2 minutes until spinach wilts.
4. **Whisk Eggs:**
   - While veggies are cooking, whisk eggs in a bowl and season with salt and pepper.
5. **Pour Eggs Over Veggies:**
   - Pour the whisked eggs over the sautéed veggies in the pan.
6. **Cook and Fold:**
   - Allow the eggs to set slightly, then gently lift the edges with a spatula, letting any uncooked egg flow underneath.

- Once the omelet is mostly set, sprinkle feta cheese over one half and fold the other half over the filling.

7. **Finish Cooking:**
   - Cook for an additional 1-2 minutes until the eggs are fully cooked but still moist.

8. **Serve:**
   - Slide the omelet onto a plate and serve immediately.

Tips and Variations:

- Experiment with different veggies and cheeses based on your preferences.
- For added protein, include diced turkey or chicken.
- Top with fresh herbs like parsley or chives for extra flavor.

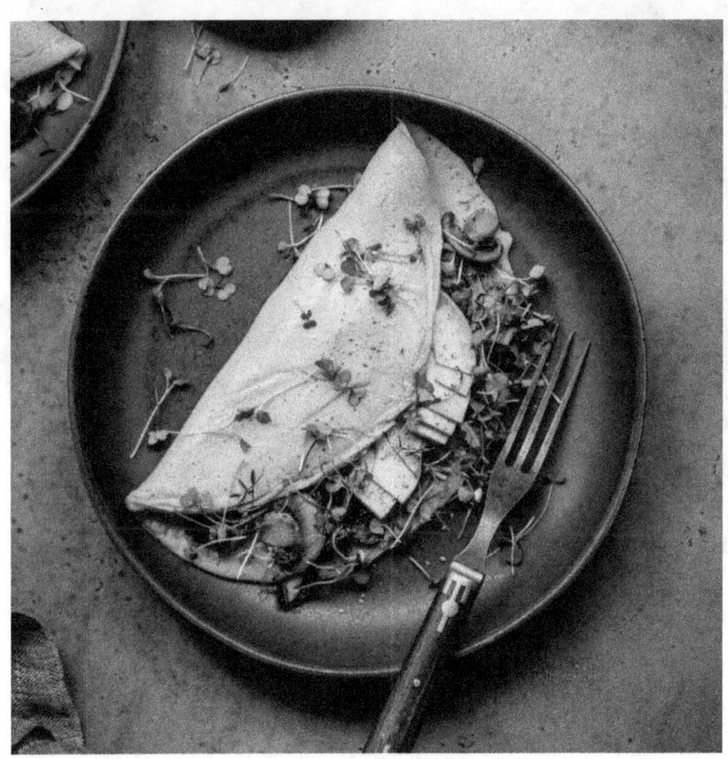

Smoothie Sensation

Preparation Time: 5 minutes
Yield: 1 serving

Ingredients:

- 1 cup kale or spinach leaves
- 1/2 banana, frozen
- 1/2 cup mixed berries (blueberries, strawberries, raspberries)
- 1/2 cup Greek yogurt
- 1/2 cup almond milk
- Ice cubes (optional)

Procedure:

1. **Prepare *Ingredients*:**
   - Wash and prepare the kale or spinach leaves.
2. **Blend:**
   - In a blender, combine kale or spinach, frozen banana, mixed berries, Greek yogurt, and almond milk.
3. **Blend Until Smooth:**
   - Blend until smooth and creamy. Add ice cubes if a colder consistency is desired.
4. **Serve:**
   - Pour the smoothie into a glass and enjoy immediately.

Tips and Variations:

- Add a scoop of protein powder for an extra protein boost.
- Adjust the thickness by adding more or less almond milk.
- Sweeten with a drizzle of honey if desired.

Cherry Almond Breakfast Quinoa

Preparation Time: 5 minutes
Cooking Time: 15 minutes
Yield: 2 servings

Ingredients:

- 1/2 cup quinoa, rinsed
- 1 cup unsweetened almond milk
- 1 cup fresh cherries, pitted and halved
- 2 tablespoons sliced almonds
- 1 tablespoon honey
- A pinch of cinnamon

Procedure:

1. **Prepare *Ingredients*:**
   - Rinse quinoa, pit and halve cherries, and measure out sliced almonds.
2. **Cook Quinoa:**
   - In a saucepan, combine quinoa and almond milk. Bring to a boil, then reduce heat to low, cover, and simmer for 12-15 minutes until quinoa is cooked and liquid is absorbed.
3. **Add Cherries and Almonds:**
   - Gently fold in fresh cherries and sliced almonds.
4. **Sweeten and Spice:**
   - Drizzle honey over the quinoa and sprinkle with a pinch of cinnamon. Mix well.
5. **Serve:**
   - Divide the Cherry Almond Breakfast Quinoa into bowls and serve warm.

Tips and Variations:

- Replace almond milk with your preferred milk alternative.
- Top with a dollop of Greek yogurt for added creaminess.
- Experiment with different fruits like peaches or berries.

Egg and Spinach Breakfast Wrap

Preparation Time: 10 minutes
Cooking Time: 5 minutes
Yield: 1 serving

Ingredients:

- 2 large eggs
- 1 cup fresh spinach, chopped
- 1/4 cup cherry tomatoes, diced
- 1 whole grain wrap
- 1 tablespoon feta cheese, crumbled
- Salt and pepper to taste
- 1 teaspoon olive oil

Procedure:

1. **Prepare *Ingredients*:**
   - Chop fresh spinach, dice cherry tomatoes, and crumble feta cheese.
2. **Whisk Eggs:**
   - In a bowl, whisk the eggs and season with salt and pepper.
3. **Cook Spinach and Tomatoes:**
   - Heat olive oil in a skillet over medium heat.
   - Add chopped spinach and diced tomatoes, sauté until spinach wilts.
4. **Add Eggs:**
   - Pour whisked eggs over the spinach and tomatoes.
5. **Scramble and Assemble:**
   - Scramble the eggs with the vegetables until fully cooked.
   - Place the cooked eggs in the center of a whole grain wrap.
6. **Top with Feta:**
   - Sprinkle crumbled feta cheese over the eggs.
7. **Wrap and Serve:**

- Fold the sides of the wrap over the eggs, creating a
  burrito-like shape.
- Serve immediately.

Tips and Variations:

- Customize with additional veggies like bell peppers or
  mushrooms.
- Experiment with different herbs or spices for added flavor.
- Serve with a side of salsa or hot sauce for extra kick.

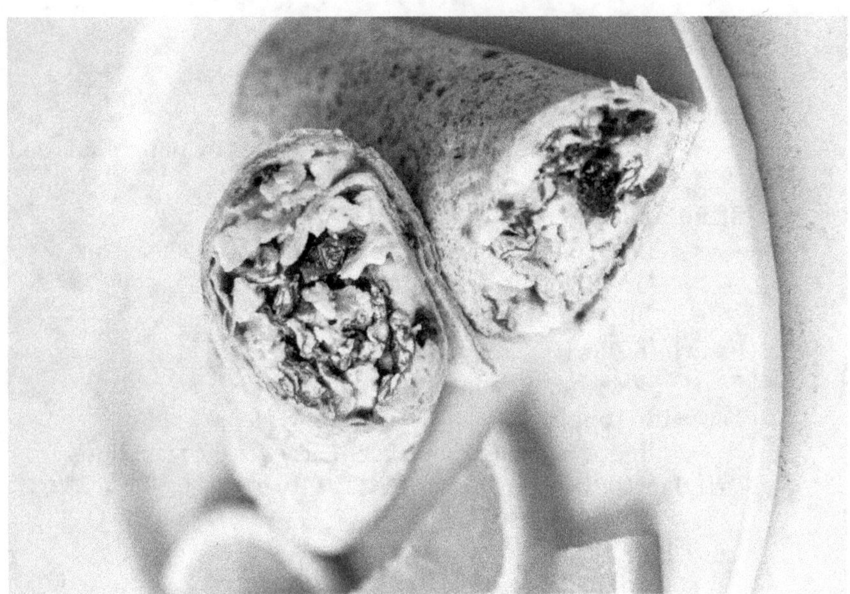

Berry Protein Smoothie Bowl

Preparation Time: 5 minutes
Yield: 1 serving

Ingredients:

- 1 cup mixed berries (strawberries, blueberries, raspberries)
- 1/2 banana, frozen
- 1/2 cup Greek yogurt
- 1 scoop protein powder (optional)
- 1/4 cup granola
- 1 tablespoon chia seeds
- Honey for drizzling (optional)

Procedure:

1. **Prepare *Ingredients*:**
   - Wash berries, slice banana, and measure out granola and chia seeds.
2. **Blend Smoothie:**
   - In a blender, combine mixed berries, frozen banana, Greek yogurt, and protein powder if using.
   - Blend until smooth.
3. **Pour into Bowl:**
   - Pour the smoothie into a bowl.
4. **Top with Toppings:**
   - Sprinkle granola and chia seeds over the smoothie.
5. **Drizzle with Honey:**
   - Drizzle honey over the top if desired.
6. **Serve and Enjoy:**
   - Serve immediately with a spoon.

Tips and Variations:

- Customize with your favorite fruits and toppings.
- Add a tablespoon of nut butter for extra creaminess.
- Experiment with different flavors of protein powder.

Sweet Potato and Black Bean Breakfast Burrito

Preparation Time: 15 minutes
Cooking Time: 15 minutes
Yield: 2 servings

Ingredients:

- 1 medium sweet potato, peeled and diced
- 1 can (15 oz) black beans, drained and rinsed
- 1/2 teaspoon cumin
- 1/2 teaspoon paprika
- Salt and pepper to taste
- 4 whole grain tortillas
- 4 eggs, scrambled
- Salsa and avocado for topping

Procedure:

1. **Prepare *Ingredients*:**
   - Peel and dice the sweet potato, drain and rinse the black beans, and scramble the eggs.
2. **Cook Sweet Potatoes:**
   - In a skillet, sauté diced sweet potatoes until tender. Add cumin, paprika, salt, and pepper.
3. **Add Black Beans:**
   - Stir in black beans and cook until heated through.
4. **Scramble Eggs:**
   - In a separate pan, scramble the eggs until cooked.
5. **Assemble Burritos:**
   - Warm tortillas and divide sweet potato and black bean mixture among them.
   - Top with scrambled eggs.
6. **Add Toppings:**
   - Add salsa and slices of avocado.
7. **Fold and Serve:**
   - Fold the sides of the tortilla over the filling, creating a burrito.
   - Serve immediately.

Tips and Variations:

- Customize with additional veggies like bell peppers or onions.
- For added heat, include jalapeños or a dash of hot sauce.
- Top with a dollop of Greek yogurt for extra creaminess.

These recipes adhere to the Dash Diet principles, providing nutrient-dense and flavorful options for a wholesome breakfast. Adjust portion sizes based on individual dietary needs.

Baked Lemon Herb Chicken

Preparation Time: 10 minutes
Cooking Time: 25 minutes
Yield: 2 servings

Ingredients:

- 2 boneless, skinless chicken breasts
- 1 lemon, juiced and zester
- 2 tablespoons olive oil
- 2 cloves garlic, minced
- 1 teaspoon dried oregano
- 1 teaspoon dried thyme
- Salt and pepper to taste
- Fresh parsley for garnish

Procedure:

1. **Preheat Oven:**
   - Preheat the oven to 400°F (200°C).
2. **Marinate Chicken:**
   - In a bowl, mix together lemon juice, lemon zest, olive oil, minced garlic, oregano, thyme, salt, and pepper.
3. **Coat Chicken:**

- Coat chicken breasts with the lemon herb mixture, ensuring they are well covered.

4. **Bake:**
   - Place the marinated chicken breasts in a baking dish and bake for 20-25 minutes or until the internal temperature reaches 165°F (74°C).

5. **Garnish and Serve:**
   - Garnish with fresh parsley and serve with a side of steamed vegetables or a green salad.

Tips and Variations:

- Add a touch of honey to the marinade for a hint of sweetness.
- Serve with quinoa or brown rice for a complete meal.
- Experiment with different herb combinations based on your preferences.

Greek Chickpea Salad

Preparation Time: 15 minutes
Yield: 4 servings

Ingredients:

- 2 cans (15 oz each) chickpeas, drained and rinsed
- 1 cucumber, diced
- 1 cup cherry tomatoes, halved
- 1/2 cup Kalamata olives, sliced
- 1/2 cup feta cheese, crumbled
- 1/4 cup red onion, finely chopped
- 3 tablespoons extra-virgin olive oil
- 2 tablespoons red wine vinegar
- 1 teaspoon dried oregano
- Salt and pepper to taste

Procedure:

1. **Combine *Ingredients*:**
   - In a large bowl, combine chickpeas, cucumber, cherry tomatoes, olives, feta cheese, and red onion.
2. **Prepare Dressing:**
   - In a small bowl, whisk together olive oil, red wine vinegar, dried oregano, salt, and pepper.
3. **Toss and Coat:**
   - Pour the dressing over the salad and toss until well coated.
4. **Chill and Serve:**
   - Refrigerate for at least 30 minutes before serving. Serve chilled.

Tips and Variations:

- Add chopped fresh parsley for an extra burst of flavor.
- For a heartier meal, serve over a bed of mixed greens.
- Customize with additional veggies like bell peppers or artichoke hearts.

Minestrone Vegetable Soup

Preparation Time: 15 minutes
Cooking Time: 30 minutes
Yield: 6 servings

Ingredients:

- 1 tablespoon olive oil
- 1 onion, diced
- 2 carrots, diced
- 2 celery stalks, diced
- 3 cloves garlic, minced
- 1 can (15 oz) diced tomatoes
- 1 can (15 oz) kidney beans, drained and rinsed
- 1 zucchini, diced
- 1 cup green beans, chopped
- 1 cup whole wheat pasta
- 6 cups vegetable broth
- 1 teaspoon dried oregano
- 1 teaspoon dried basil
- Salt and pepper to taste
- Parmesan cheese for serving (optional)

Procedure:

1. **Saute Aromatics:**
    - In a large pot, heat olive oil over medium heat. Add diced onion, carrots, celery, and garlic. Saute until vegetables are softened.
2. **Add Tomatoes and Beans:**
    - Stir in diced tomatoes, kidney beans, zucchini, and green beans.
3. **Pour Broth:**
    - Pour in vegetable broth and add whole wheat pasta.
4. **Season:**
    - Season with dried oregano, dried basil, salt, and pepper. Bring to a simmer.
5. **Simmer and Serve:**

- Simmer for 20-25 minutes until pasta and vegetables are cooked. Adjust seasoning if needed.

6. **Serve:**
   - Ladle into bowls and optionally sprinkle with Parmesan cheese before serving.

Tips and Variations:

- Substitute whole wheat pasta with quinoa for a gluten-free option.
- Add a handful of fresh spinach just before serving.
- Experiment with different herbs like thyme or rosemary.

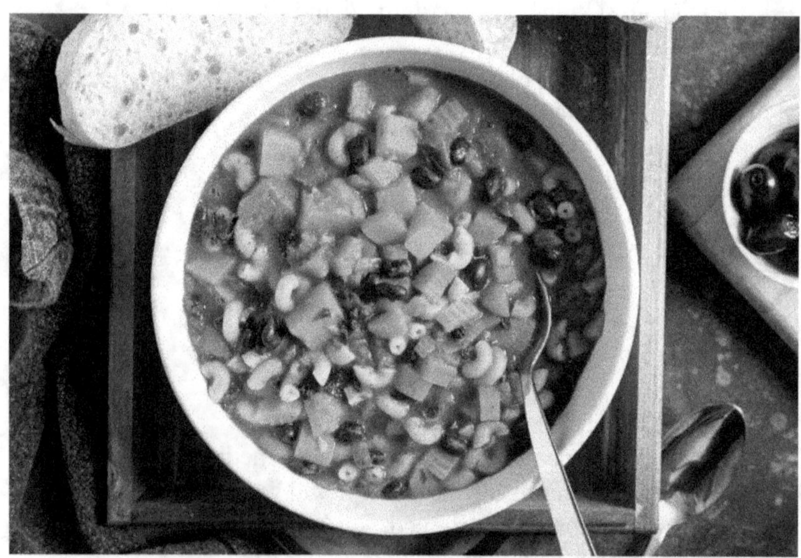

Turkey and Avocado Wrap

Preparation Time: 10 minutes
Yield: 2 servings

Ingredients:

- 1/2 lb turkey breast, sliced
- 2 whole grain wraps
- 1 avocado, sliced
- 1 cup lettuce, shredded
- 1 tomato, sliced
- 2 tablespoons Dijon mustard
- Salt and pepper to taste

Procedure:

1. **Assemble Wraps:**
   - Lay out the whole grain wraps and divide sliced turkey between them.
2. **Layer *Ingredients*:**
   - Top with avocado slices, shredded lettuce, and tomato slices.
3. **Season and Dress:**
   - Season with salt and pepper and spread Dijon mustard over the ***ingredients***.
4. **Wrap and Serve:**
   - Roll the wraps, folding in the sides, to create a tight wrap.
5. **Slice and Enjoy:**
   - Slice in half and enjoy immediately.

Tips and Variations:

- Add a slice of Swiss or cheddar cheese for extra flavor.
- Drizzle with balsamic glaze for a tangy twist.
- Incorporate pickles or red onion for added crunch.

Apple Cinnamon Overnight Oats

Preparation Time: 10 minutes (plus overnight chilling)
Yield: 1 serving

Ingredients:

- 1/2 cup rolled oats
- 1/2 cup unsweetened almond milk
- 1/2 apple, diced
- 1 tablespoon chopped walnuts
- 1 teaspoon chia seeds
- 1/2 teaspoon cinnamon
- 1 teaspoon honey (optional)

Procedure:

1. **Combine *Ingredients*:**
   - In a jar or container, mix rolled oats, almond milk, diced apple, chopped walnuts, chia seeds, and cinnamon.
2. **Stir and Seal:**
   - Stir well to combine, ensuring oats are fully submerged in almond milk. Seal the jar or container.
3. **Chill Overnight:**
   - Refrigerate overnight or for at least 6 hours to allow the oats to absorb the liquid.
4. **Serve and Sweeten:**
   - In the morning, give the oats a good stir. Add a drizzle of honey if desired and enjoy.

Tips and Variations:

- Experiment with different apple varieties for varied sweetness.
- Top with a dollop of Greek yogurt for added creaminess.
- Customize with your favorite nuts or seeds.

Spinach and Mushroom Breakfast Wrap

Preparation Time: 15 minutes
Cooking Time: 5 minutes
Yield: 1 serving

Ingredients:

- 2 large eggs
- 1 cup fresh spinach, chopped
- 1/2 cup mushrooms, sliced
- 1 whole grain wrap
- 1 tablespoon feta cheese, crumbled
- Salt and pepper to taste
- 1 teaspoon olive oil

Procedure:

1. **Prepare *Ingredients*:**
   - Chop fresh spinach, slice mushrooms, and crumble feta cheese.
2. **Saute Spinach and Mushrooms:**
   - Heat olive oil in a skillet over medium heat. Add chopped spinach and sliced mushrooms. Saute until spinach wilts and mushrooms are cooked.
3. **Whisk Eggs:**
   - In a bowl, whisk the eggs and season with salt and pepper.
4. **Cook Eggs:**
   - Push the sauteed spinach and mushrooms to one side of the pan. Pour whisked eggs into the empty side.
5. **Scramble and Assemble:**
   - Scramble the eggs until fully cooked. Place the cooked eggs in the center of the whole grain wrap.
6. **Top with Feta:**
   - Sprinkle crumbled feta cheese over the eggs.
7. **Wrap and Serve:**
   - Fold the sides of the wrap over the eggs, creating a burrito-like shape. Serve immediately.

Tips and Variations:

- Add diced tomatoes or bell peppers for extra freshness.
- Incorporate your favorite herbs or spices.
- Serve with a side of salsa for added flavor.

Peach and Walnut Breakfast Parfait

Preparation Time: 10 minutes
Yield: 1 serving

Ingredients:

- 1 cup Greek yogurt
- 1 peach, sliced
- 2 tablespoons chopped walnuts
- 1 tablespoon honey
- 1/4 cup granola

Procedure:

1. **Layer Greek Yogurt:**
   - In a glass or bowl, start with a layer of Greek yogurt.
2. **Add Sliced Peaches:**
   - Top the yogurt with slices of fresh peach.
3. **Sprinkle Walnuts:**
   - Sprinkle chopped walnuts over the peaches.
4. **Drizzle with Honey:**
   - Drizzle honey over the layers.
5. **Top with Granola:**
   - Finish with a layer of granola for added crunch.
6. **Repeat Layers:**
   - Repeat the layers until the glass or bowl is filled.
7. **Serve and Enjoy:**
   - Serve immediately and enjoy this delightful Peach and Walnut Breakfast Parfait.

Tips and Variations:

- Use flavored Greek yogurt for added sweetness.
- Experiment with different fruits based on seasonal availability.
- Substitute the honey with maple syrup for a different flavor profile.

Protein-Packed Cottage Cheese Bowl

Preparation Time: 5 minutes
Yield: 1 serving

Ingredients:

- 1 cup low-fat cottage cheese
- 1/2 cup mixed berries (strawberries, blueberries, raspberries)
- 1 tablespoon sunflower seeds
- 1 tablespoon honey

Procedure:

1. **Combine Cottage Cheese:**
   - In a bowl, combine low-fat cottage cheese.
2. **Add Mixed Berries:**
   - Top the cottage cheese with a mix of fresh berries.
3. **Sprinkle Sunflower Seeds:**
   - Sprinkle sunflower seeds over the berries.
4. **Drizzle with Honey:**
   - Drizzle honey over the entire bowl.
5. **Serve and Enjoy:**
   - Serve immediately, savoring the protein-packed goodness of this cottage cheese bowl.

Tips and Variations:

- Add a dash of cinnamon for extra flavor.
- Incorporate a scoop of protein powder for an additional protein boost.
- Use different seeds like chia seeds or flaxseeds.

Quinoa and Vegetable Stuffed Bell Peppers

Preparation Time: 15 minutes
Cooking Time: 30 minutes
Yield: 4 servings

Ingredients:

- 4 bell peppers, halved and seeds removed
- 1 cup cooked quinoa
- 1 can (15 oz) black beans, drained and rinsed
- 1 cup cherry tomatoes, diced
- 1 cup corn kernels (fresh or frozen)
- 1/2 cup red onion, finely chopped
- 1 teaspoon cumin
- 1 teaspoon chili powder
- Salt and pepper to taste
- 1 cup shredded low-fat cheddar cheese

Procedure:

1. **Preheat Oven:**
   - Preheat the oven to 375°F (190°C).
2. **Prepare Peppers:**
   - Place bell pepper halves in a baking dish.
3. **Mix Filling:**
   - In a bowl, combine cooked quinoa, black beans, cherry tomatoes, corn, red onion, cumin, chili powder, salt, and pepper.
4. **Stuff Peppers:**
   - Fill each bell pepper half with the quinoa and vegetable mixture.
5. **Top with Cheese:**
   - Sprinkle shredded cheddar cheese over the stuffed peppers.
6. **Bake:**
   - Bake in the preheated oven for 25-30 minutes or until peppers are tender and cheese is melted and bubbly.
7. **Serve:**

- Remove from the oven and serve immediately.

Tips and Variations:

- Drizzle with salsa or Greek yogurt before serving.
- Add diced avocado for extra creaminess.
- Experiment with different colored bell peppers for visual appeal.

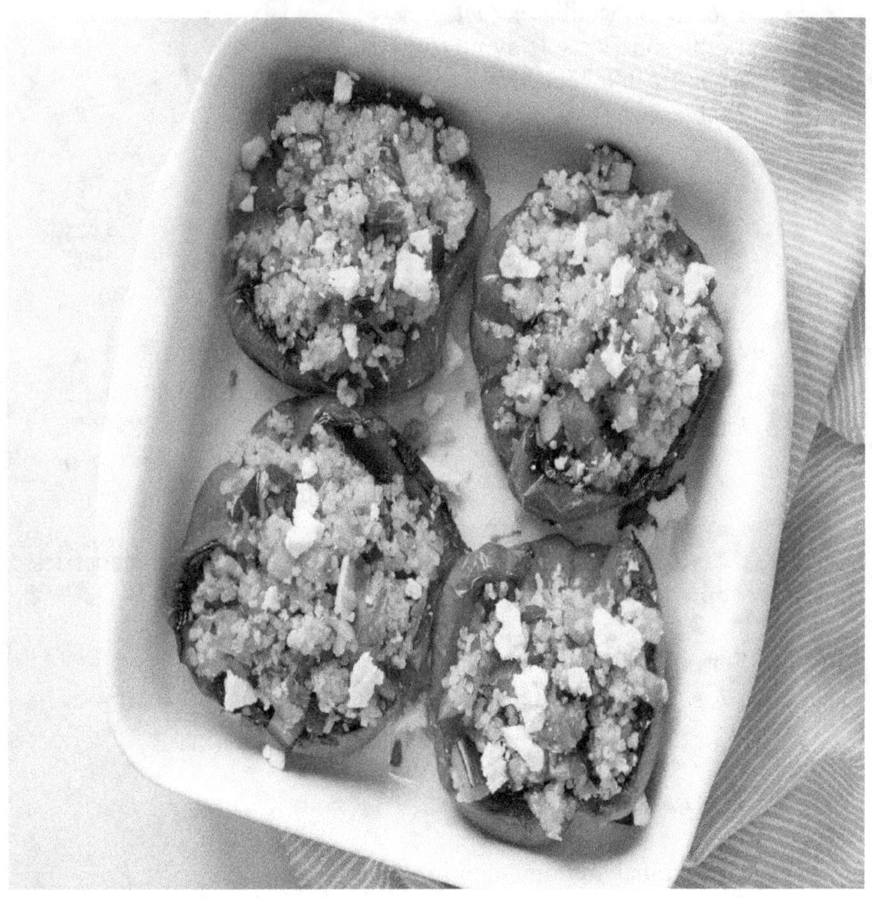

Blueberry Almond Chia Pudding

Preparation Time: 10 minutes (plus chilling time)
Yield: 2 servings

Ingredients:

- 1/2 cup chia seeds
- 2 cups unsweetened almond milk
- 1 teaspoon vanilla extract
- 1 tablespoon maple syrup (optional)
- 1 cup fresh blueberries
- 2 tablespoons sliced almonds

Procedure:

1. **Mix Chia Pudding Base:**
    - In a bowl, combine chia seeds, almond milk, vanilla extract, and maple syrup if using.
2. **Stir Well:**
    - Stir well to ensure chia seeds are evenly distributed.
3. **Chill:**
    - Cover the bowl and refrigerate for at least 4 hours or overnight to allow the chia pudding to set.
4. **Layer with Blueberries:**
    - Once set, layer the chia pudding with fresh blueberries.
5. **Top with Almonds:**
    - Sprinkle sliced almonds over the blueberries.
6. **Serve:**
    - Serve chilled and enjoy this nutritious Blueberry Almond Chia Pudding.

Tips and Variations:

- Add a pinch of cinnamon for extra flavor.
- Substitute almond milk with your preferred milk alternative.
- Customize with other berries like strawberries or raspberries.

Turkey and Quinoa Stuffed Zucchini Boats

Preparation Time: 20 minutes
Cooking Time: 25 minutes
Yield: 4 servings

Ingredients:

- 2 large zucchini, halved lengthwise
- 1 cup cooked quinoa
- 1/2 lb lean ground turkey
- 1/2 cup onion, finely chopped
- 1/2 cup bell pepper, diced
- 1 clove garlic, minced
- 1 can (15 oz) diced tomatoes, drained
- 1 teaspoon dried oregano
- 1 teaspoon dried basil
- Salt and pepper to taste
- 1/2 cup shredded mozzarella cheese

Procedure:

1. **Preheat Oven:**
   - Preheat the oven to 375°F (190°C).
2. **Prepare Zucchini Boats:**
   - Scoop out the centers of the zucchini halves, creating boat-shaped shells. Reserve the scooped zucchini.
3. **Cook Turkey and Vegetables:**
   - In a skillet, cook ground turkey, onion, bell pepper, and garlic until turkey is browned and vegetables are softened.
4. **Add Remaining *Ingredients*:**
   - Stir in cooked quinoa, diced tomatoes, dried oregano, dried basil, salt, and pepper. Add the reserved scooped zucchini.
5. **Fill Zucchini Boats:**
   - Fill each zucchini boat with the turkey and quinoa mixture.
6. **Top with Cheese:**

- Sprinkle shredded mozzarella cheese over the stuffed zucchini.

7. **Bake:**
   - Bake in the preheated oven for 20-25 minutes or until zucchini is tender and cheese is melted and golden.

8. **Serve:**
   - Remove from the oven and serve immediately.

Tips and Variations:

- Garnish with fresh herbs like parsley before serving.
- Drizzle with balsamic glaze for added flavor.
- Include diced tomatoes or salsa for a burst of freshness.

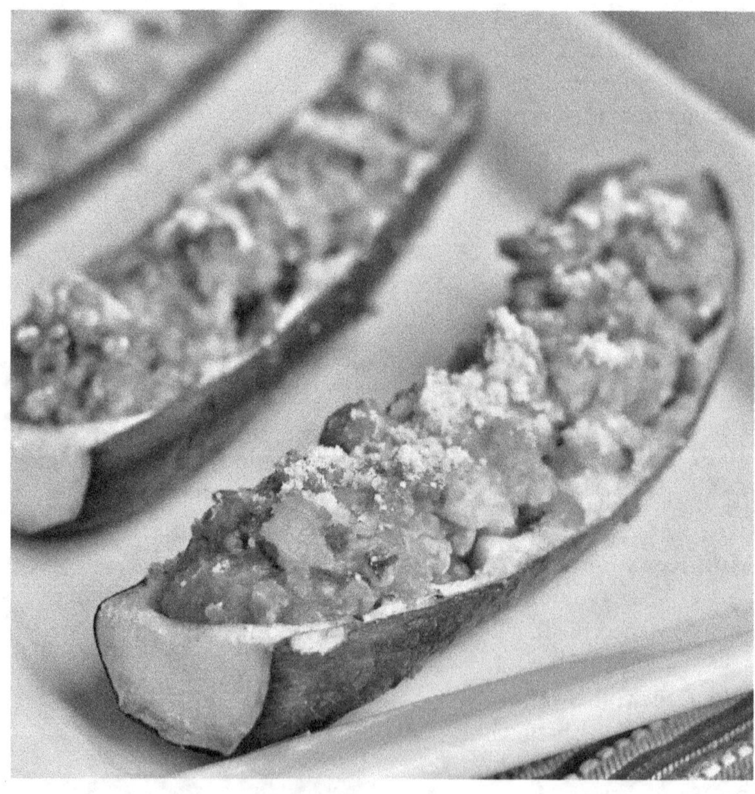

Salmon and Asparagus Foil Packets

Preparation Time: 15 minutes
Cooking Time: 20 minutes
Yield: 2 servings

Ingredients:

- 2 salmon fillets
- 1 bunch asparagus, trimmed
- 1 lemon, thinly sliced
- 2 tablespoons olive oil
- 2 cloves garlic, minced
- 1 teaspoon dried dill
- Salt and pepper to taste

Procedure:

1. **Preheat Oven:**
   - Preheat the oven to 400°F (200°C).
2. **Prepare Foil Packets:**
   - Place each salmon fillet on a piece of aluminum foil. Arrange asparagus around the salmon.
3. **Season and Drizzle:**
   - In a bowl, mix together olive oil, minced garlic, dried dill, salt, and pepper. Drizzle the mixture over the salmon and asparagus.
4. **Top with Lemon Slices:**
   - Place lemon slices over the salmon fillets.
5. **Seal Packets:**
   - Fold the foil over the salmon and asparagus, sealing the edges to create packets.
6. **Bake:**
   - Bake in the preheated oven for 18-20 minutes or until salmon is cooked through.
7. **Serve:**
   - Carefully open the foil packets and serve immediately.

Tips and Variations:

- Garnish with fresh parsley or chopped green onions before serving.
- Experiment with different herbs like thyme or rosemary.
- Include cherry tomatoes for extra juiciness.

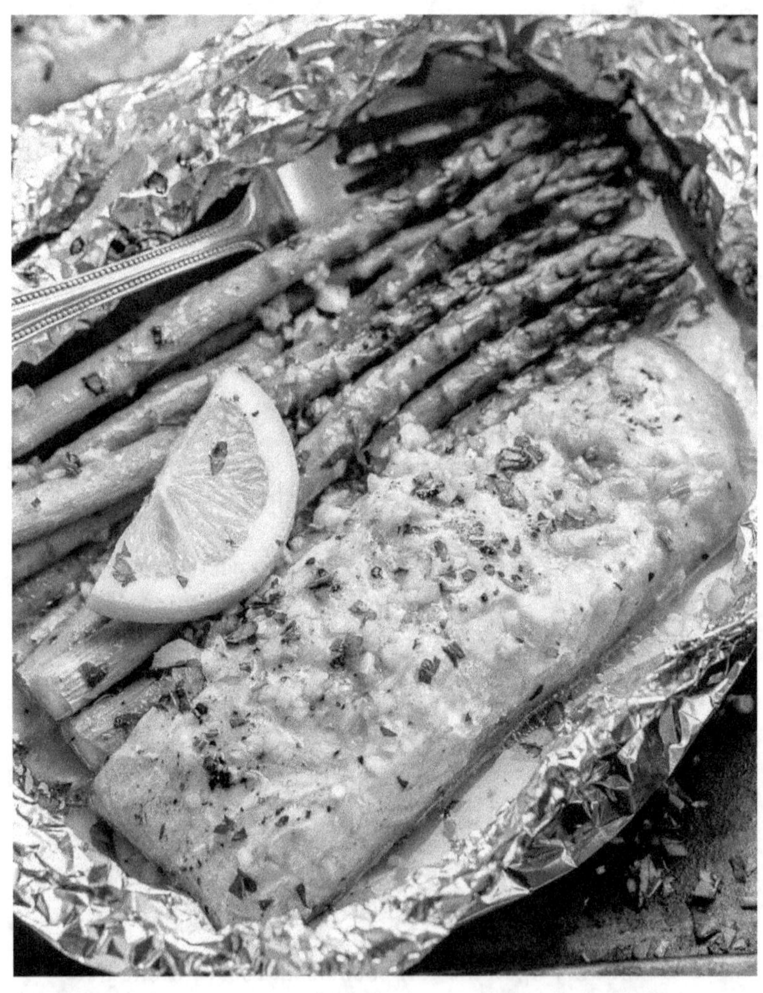

Avocado and Tomato Breakfast Toast

Preparation Time: 10 minutes
Yield: 2 servings

Ingredients:

- 4 slices whole grain bread, toasted
- 1 large avocado, mashed
- 1 cup cherry tomatoes, halved
- 1 tablespoon olive oil
- 1 teaspoon balsamic glaze (optional)
- Salt and pepper to taste
- Red pepper flakes for a spicy kick (optional)

Procedure:

1. **Toast Bread:**
   - Toast the slices of whole grain bread until golden brown.
2. **Mash Avocado:**
   - In a bowl, mash the avocado with a fork and season with salt and pepper.
3. **Assemble Toasts:**
   - Spread the mashed avocado evenly over each slice of toasted bread.
4. **Top with Tomatoes:**
   - Arrange halved cherry tomatoes over the mashed avocado.
5. **Drizzle with Olive Oil:**
   - Drizzle olive oil over the tomatoes. Add balsamic glaze if using.
6. **Season and Serve:**
   - Season with additional salt and pepper to taste. Sprinkle red pepper flakes for a spicy kick.
7. **Serve:**
   - Serve immediately and enjoy this simple and satisfying Avocado and Tomato Breakfast Toast.

Tips and Variations:

- Add a sprinkle of feta cheese for a tangy twist.
- Garnish with fresh basil or cilantro for added flavor.
- Include a poached or fried egg on top for extra protein.

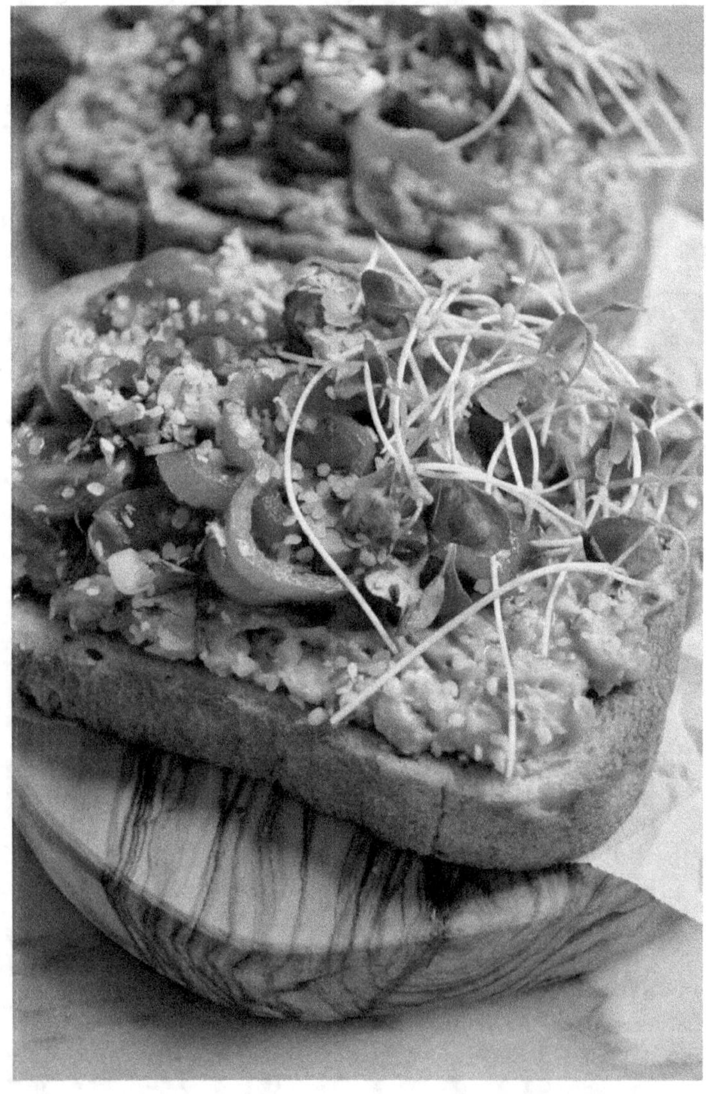

Chickpea and Vegetable Stir-Fry

Preparation Time: 15 minutes
Cooking Time: 15 minutes
Yield: 4 servings

Ingredients:

- 2 tablespoons olive oil
- 1 onion, sliced
- 2 bell peppers, thinly sliced
- 1 zucchini, sliced
- 1 cup cherry tomatoes, halved
- 2 cups cooked chickpeas (canned or cooked from dry)
- 3 cups baby spinach
- 2 tablespoons soy sauce
- 1 tablespoon sesame oil
- 1 teaspoon grated ginger
- 2 cloves garlic, minced
- Sesame seeds for garnish (optional)

Procedure:

1. **Saute Vegetables:**
   - In a wok or large skillet, heat olive oil over medium-high heat. Add sliced onion, bell peppers, and zucchini. Stir-fry until vegetables are tender-crisp.
2. **Add Cherry Tomatoes:**
   - Add cherry tomatoes to the stir-fry and cook for an additional 2 minutes.
3. **Incorporate Chickpeas:**
   - Stir in cooked chickpeas and cook until heated through.
4. **Fold in Spinach:**
   - Add baby spinach to the stir-fry and cook until wilted.
5. **Prepare Sauce:**
   - In a small bowl, whisk together soy sauce, sesame oil, grated ginger, and minced garlic.
6. **Pour Sauce and Toss:**

- Pour the sauce over the stir-fried vegetables and chickpeas. Toss everything together until well coated.

7. **Garnish and Serve:**
   - Garnish with sesame seeds if desired. Serve this Chickpea and Vegetable Stir-Fry over brown rice or quinoa.

Tips and Variations:

- Customize with your favorite stir-fry vegetables.
- Drizzle with a bit of sriracha for extra heat.
- Top with chopped green onions for freshness.

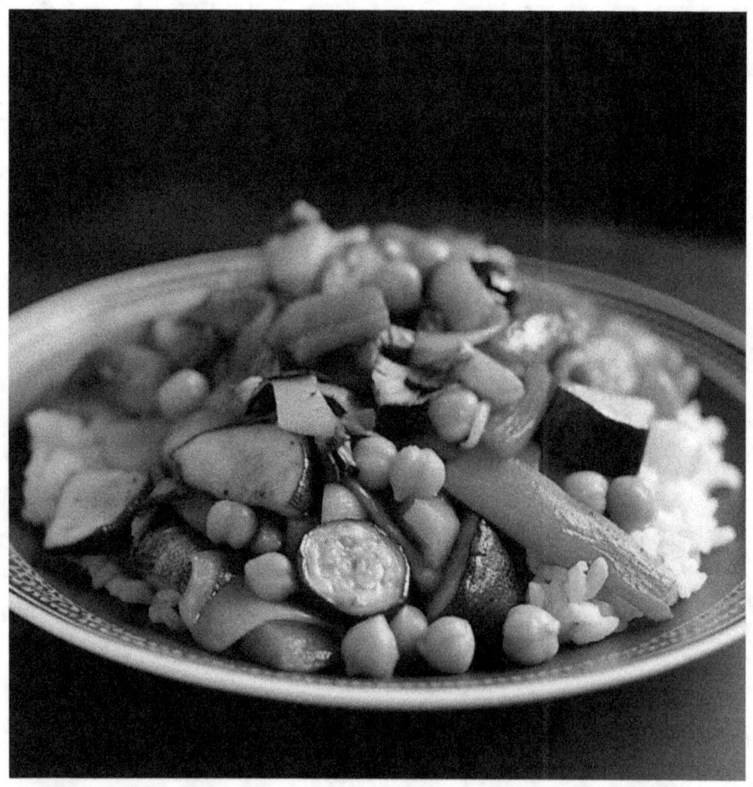

Lunch delight

Grilled Chicken Salad with Balsamic Vinaigrette

Preparation Time: 15 minutes
Cooking Time: 10 minutes
Yield: 2 servings

Ingredients:

- 2 boneless, skinless chicken breasts
- Salt and black pepper to taste
- 6 cups mixed salad greens
- 1 cup cherry tomatoes, halved
- 1 cucumber, sliced
- 1/4 cup red onion, thinly sliced
- 1/3 cup feta cheese, crumbled
- 2 tablespoons balsamic vinaigrette dressing

Procedure:

1. **Grill Chicken:**
   - Season chicken breasts with salt and black pepper. Grill until fully cooked, about 5 minutes per side. Let them rest for a few minutes before slicing.
2. **Prepare Salad Base:**
   - In a large bowl, combine mixed salad greens, cherry tomatoes, cucumber slices, and thinly sliced red onion.
3. **Slice Chicken:**
   - Slice the grilled chicken breasts into thin strips.
4. **Assemble Salad:**
   - Add the sliced chicken on top of the salad base. Sprinkle crumbled feta cheese over the salad.
5. **Drizzle Dressing:**
   - Drizzle balsamic vinaigrette dressing over the salad. Toss gently to combine.

6. **Serve:**
   - Divide the salad into plates and serve immediately.

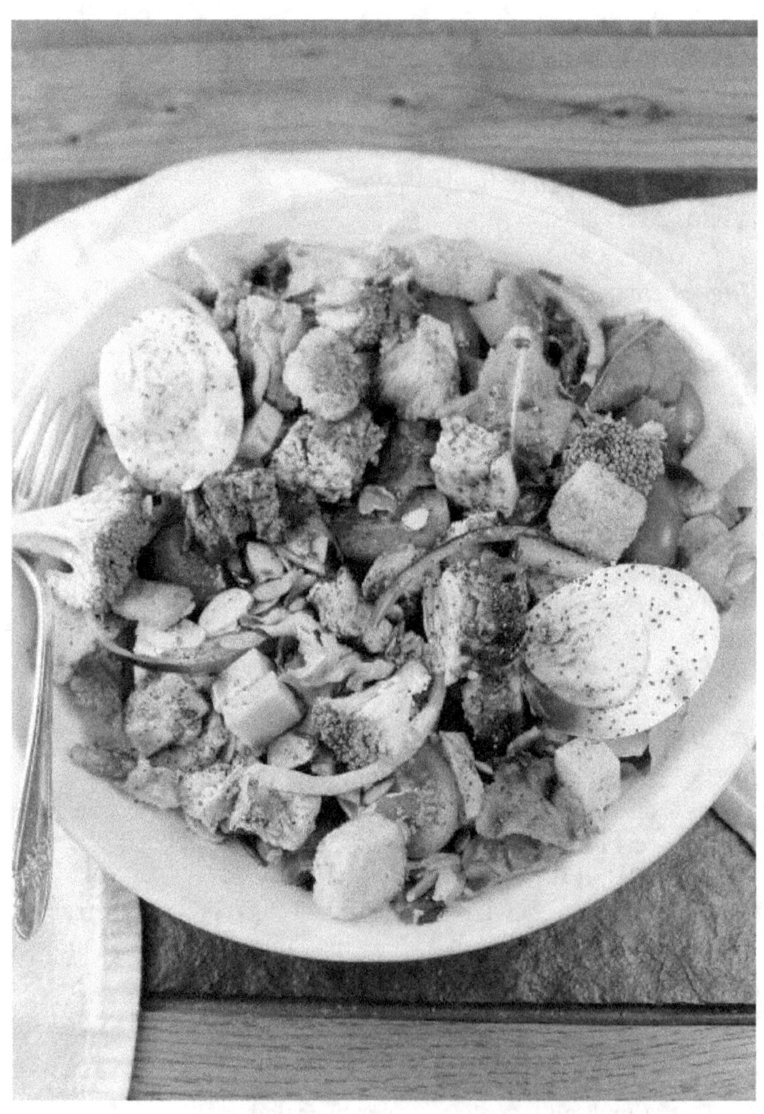

Quinoa and Black Bean Stuffed Bell Peppers

Preparation Time: 20 minutes
Cooking Time: 30 minutes
Yield: 4 servings

Ingredients:

- 4 large bell peppers, halved and seeds removed
- 1 cup cooked quinoa
- 1 can (15 oz) black beans, drained and rinsed
- 1 cup corn kernels (fresh or frozen)
- 1 cup cherry tomatoes, diced
- 1/2 cup red onion, finely chopped
- 1 teaspoon cumin
- 1 teaspoon chili powder
- Salt and pepper to taste
- 1 cup shredded low-fat cheddar cheese

Procedure:

1. **Preheat Oven:**
   - Preheat the oven to 375°F (190°C).
2. **Prepare Peppers:**
   - Place bell pepper halves in a baking dish.
3. **Mix Filling:**
   - In a bowl, combine cooked quinoa, black beans, cherry tomatoes, corn, red onion, cumin, chili powder, salt, and pepper.
4. **Stuff Peppers:**
   - Fill each bell pepper half with the quinoa and vegetable mixture.
5. **Top with Cheese:**
   - Sprinkle shredded cheddar cheese over the stuffed peppers.
6. **Bake:**
   - Bake in the preheated oven for 25-30 minutes or until peppers are tender and cheese is melted and bubbly.
7. **Serve:** Remove from the oven and serve immediately.

Turkey and Veggie Wrap with Whole Wheat Tortilla

Preparation Time: 15 minutes
Yield: 2 servings

Ingredients:

- 4 whole wheat tortillas
- 1/2 lb lean ground turkey
- 1 teaspoon olive oil
- 1 teaspoon taco seasoning
- 1 cup mixed salad greens
- 1 tomato, diced
- 1/2 cup black beans, drained and rinsed
- 1/2 cup corn kernels (fresh or frozen)
- 1/4 cup Greek yogurt (optional)
- Salsa for serving

Procedure:

1. **Cook Turkey:**
   - In a skillet, heat olive oil over medium heat. Add ground turkey and cook until browned. Season with taco seasoning.
2. **Prepare Wraps:**
   - Warm the whole wheat tortillas. Lay them flat on a clean surface.
3. **Assemble Wraps:**
   - Divide the cooked turkey among the tortillas. Top with mixed salad greens, diced tomatoes, black beans, and corn.
4. **Add Greek Yogurt (Optional):**
   - If using Greek yogurt, drizzle a little over the filling.
5. **Fold and Serve:**
   - Fold the sides of the tortillas and roll them up to form wraps. Serve with salsa on the side.

Salmon and Avocado Sushi Bowls

Preparation Time: 20 minutes
Cooking Time: 10 minutes
Yield: 2 servings

Ingredients:

- 1 cup brown rice, cooked
- 2 salmon fillets
- 1 avocado, sliced
- 1 cucumber, julienned
- 1 carrot, julienned
- 2 tablespoons soy sauce
- 1 tablespoon rice vinegar
- 1 teaspoon sesame oil
- 1 teaspoon sesame seeds
- Nori sheets, shredded (optional)

Procedure:

1. **Cook Salmon:**
   - Grill or bake the salmon fillets until fully cooked. Once cooked, flake the salmon into bite-sized pieces.
2. **Prepare Rice:**
   - Cook brown rice according to package instructions.
3. **Assemble Bowls:**
   - Divide cooked rice among two bowls. Top with flaked salmon, sliced avocado, julienned cucumber, and julienned carrot.
4. **Make Sauce:**
   - In a small bowl, whisk together soy sauce, rice vinegar, sesame oil, and sesame seeds.
5. **Drizzle Sauce:**
   - Drizzle the sauce over the sushi bowls.
6. **Optional: Add Nori Sheets:**
   - If using nori sheets, shred them and sprinkle over the bowls.

7. **Serve:** Toss the *ingredients* in each bowl gently and serve
   immediately.

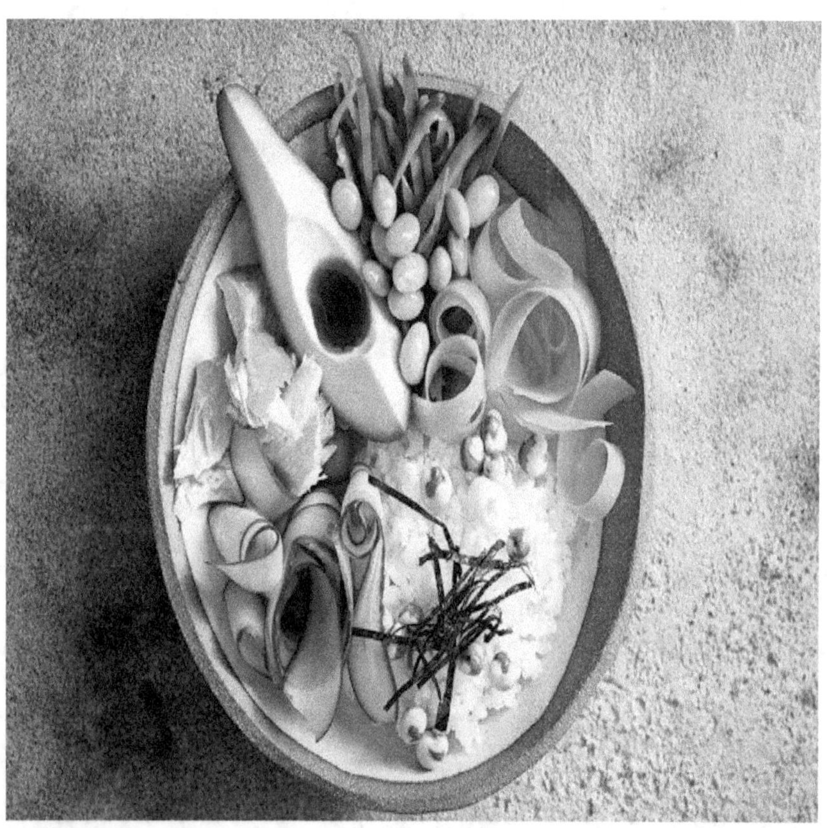

Lentil and Vegetable Soup

Preparation Time: 15 minutes
Cooking Time: 30 minutes
Yield: 4 servings

Ingredients:

- 1 cup dry green lentils, rinsed
- 1 onion, diced
- 2 carrots, sliced
- 2 celery stalks, sliced
- 3 cloves garlic, minced
- 1 can (15 oz) diced tomatoes
- 6 cups vegetable broth
- 1 teaspoon ground cumin
- 1 teaspoon ground coriander
- 1 teaspoon smoked paprika
- Salt and pepper to taste
- Fresh parsley for garnish

Procedure:

1. **Saute Vegetables:**
   - In a large pot, sauté diced onion, sliced carrots, sliced celery, and minced garlic until vegetables are softened.
2. **Add Lentils:**
   - Add rinsed green lentils to the pot and stir.
3. **Pour Broth:**
   - Pour vegetable broth into the pot.
4. **Add Tomatoes and Spices:**
   - Add diced tomatoes, ground cumin, ground coriander, smoked paprika, salt, and pepper. Stir to combine.
5. **Simmer:**
   - Bring the soup to a boil, then reduce heat and simmer for 25-30 minutes or until lentils are tender.
6. **Adjust Seasoning:**
   - Taste and adjust seasoning as needed.
7. **Garnish and Serve:** Garnish with fresh parsley before serving.

Greek Salad with Feta and Olives

Preparation Time: 15 minutes
Yield: 2 servings

Ingredients:

- 4 cups mixed salad greens
- 1 cucumber, diced
- 1 cup cherry tomatoes, halved
- 1/2 red onion, thinly sliced
- 1/2 cup Kalamata olives, pitted
- 1/2 cup feta cheese, crumbled
- 2 tablespoons extra-virgin olive oil
- 1 tablespoon red wine vinegar
- 1 teaspoon dried oregano
- Salt and black pepper to taste

Procedure:

1. **Prepare Salad Base:**
   - In a large bowl, combine mixed salad greens, diced cucumber, cherry tomatoes, thinly sliced red onion, Kalamata olives, and crumbled feta cheese.
2. **Make Dressing:**
   - In a small bowl, whisk together extra-virgin olive oil, red wine vinegar, dried oregano, salt, and black pepper.
3. **Toss Salad:**
   - Drizzle the dressing over the salad and toss gently to coat evenly.
4. **Serve:**
   - Divide the Greek Salad into plates and serve immediately.

Shrimp and Vegetable Stir-Fry

Preparation Time: 15 minutes
Cooking Time: 10 minutes
Yield: 2 servings

Ingredients:

- 8 oz shrimp, peeled and deveined
- 2 cups broccoli florets
- 1 bell pepper, sliced
- 1 carrot, julienned
- 1 cup snap peas, trimmed
- 2 tablespoons soy sauce
- 1 tablespoon hoisin sauce
- 1 tablespoon sesame oil
- 1 teaspoon ginger, minced
- 2 cloves garlic, minced
- 2 green onions, sliced
- Sesame seeds for garnish

Procedure:

1. **Prepare Shrimp:**
   - In a wok or large skillet, heat sesame oil over medium-high heat. Add shrimp and cook until they turn pink. Remove shrimp from the wok and set aside.
2. **Stir-Fry Vegetables:**
   - In the same wok, add a bit more sesame oil if needed. Stir-fry broccoli, bell pepper, carrot, snap peas, ginger, and garlic until vegetables are tender-crisp.
3. **Combine Shrimp and Vegetables:**
   - Return cooked shrimp to the wok and toss with the vegetables.
4. **Prepare Sauce:**
   - In a small bowl, mix soy sauce and hoisin sauce. Pour the sauce over the shrimp and vegetables. Toss to coat.
5. **Garnish and Serve:**

- Garnish with sliced green onions and sesame seeds. Serve over brown rice or quinoa.

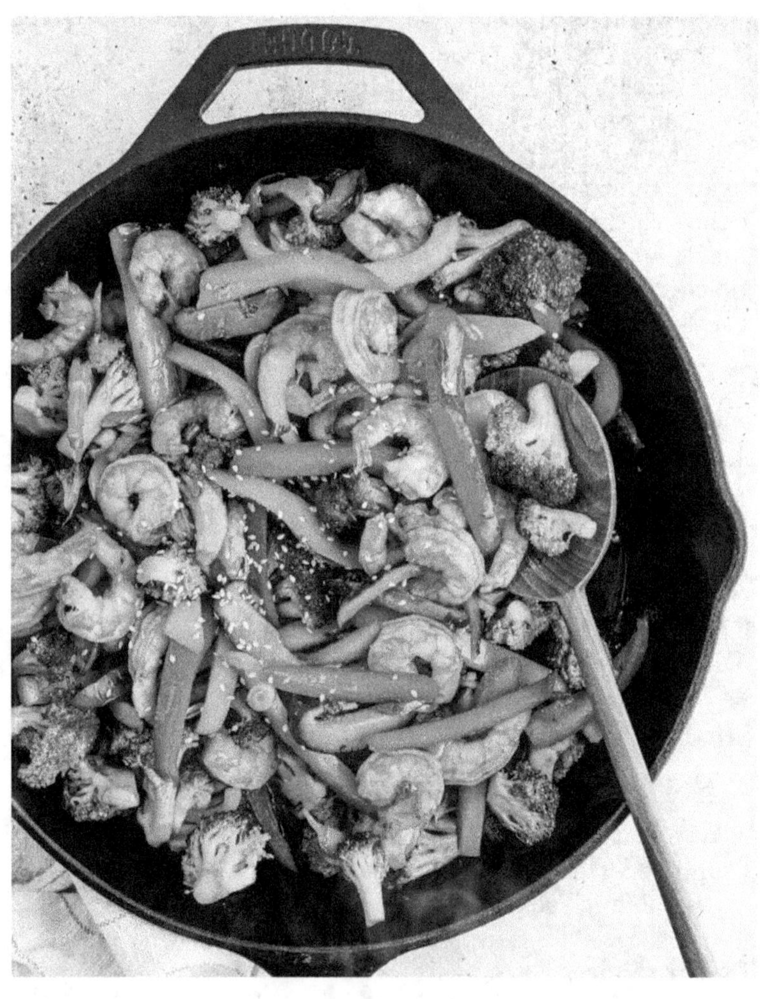

Chickpea and Spinach Salad with Lemon-Tahini Dressing

Preparation Time: 15 minutes
Yield: 2 servings

Ingredients:

- 1 can (15 oz) chickpeas, drained and rinsed
- 4 cups fresh baby spinach
- 1 cucumber, diced
- 1 cup cherry tomatoes, halved
- 1/4 cup red onion, finely chopped
- 1/4 cup fresh parsley, chopped
- 1/4 cup tahini
- 2 tablespoons lemon juice
- 1 clove garlic, minced
- 2 tablespoons water
- Salt and black pepper to taste

Procedure:

1. **Prepare Salad Base:**
   - In a large bowl, combine chickpeas, fresh baby spinach, diced cucumber, cherry tomatoes, finely chopped red onion, and chopped fresh parsley.
2. **Make Dressing:**
   - In a small bowl, whisk together tahini, lemon juice, minced garlic, water, salt, and black pepper.
3. **Toss Salad:**
   - Drizzle the lemon-tahini dressing over the salad and toss gently to coat.
4. **Serve:**
   - Divide the Chickpea and Spinach Salad into plates and serve immediately.

Mediterranean Hummus Wrap

Preparation Time: 10 minutes
Yield: 2 servings

Ingredients:

- 4 whole grain wraps
- 1 cup hummus
- 1 cup cucumber, sliced
- 1 cup cherry tomatoes, halved
- 1/2 cup Kalamata olives, pitted and sliced
- 1/2 cup feta cheese, crumbled
- 2 tablespoons fresh mint, chopped

Procedure:

1. **Warm Wraps:**
   - If desired, warm the whole grain wraps in a skillet for a few seconds on each side.
2. **Spread Hummus:**
   - Spread a generous layer of hummus over each wrap.
3. **Layer *Ingredients*:**
   - Add cucumber slices, halved cherry tomatoes, sliced Kalamata olives, crumbled feta cheese, and chopped fresh mint over the hummus.
4. **Wrap and Serve:**
   - Roll the wraps tightly, folding in the sides. Cut in half if preferred. Serve immediately.

Tuna Salad Lettuce Wraps

Preparation Time: 15 minutes
Yield: 2 servings

Ingredients:

- 1 can (5 oz) tuna, drained
- 1/4 cup Greek yogurt
- 1/4 cup celery, finely chopped
- 2 tablespoons red onion, finely chopped
- 1 tablespoon Dijon mustard
- 1 tablespoon fresh dill, chopped
- Salt and black pepper to taste
- 8 large lettuce leaves (such as iceberg or romaine)

Procedure:

1. **Prepare Tuna Salad:**
   - In a bowl, combine drained tuna, Greek yogurt, chopped celery, chopped red onion, Dijon mustard, chopped fresh dill, salt, and black pepper.
2. **Mix Well:**
   - Mix the *ingredients* until well combined.
3. **Assemble Lettuce Wraps:**
   - Spoon the tuna salad onto each lettuce leaf.
4. **Wrap and Serve:**
   - Wrap the lettuce around the tuna salad filling. Secure with toothpicks if needed. Serve immediately.

Caprese Salad with Fresh Basil

Preparation Time: 10 minutes
Yield: 2 servings

Ingredients:

- 2 large tomatoes, sliced
- 1 ball fresh mozzarella, sliced
- Fresh basil leaves
- Extra-virgin olive oil
- Balsamic glaze
- Salt and black pepper to taste

Procedure:

1. **Assemble Salad:**
   - Arrange tomato and mozzarella slices alternately on a serving plate.
2. **Add Fresh Basil:**
   - Tuck fresh basil leaves between the tomato and mozzarella slices.
3. **Drizzle with Olive Oil and Balsamic Glaze:**
   - Drizzle extra-virgin olive oil and balsamic glaze over the salad.
4. **Season:**
   - Sprinkle salt and black pepper to taste.
5. **Serve:**
   - Serve immediately as a refreshing Caprese Salad.

Sweet Potato and Chickpea Buddha Bowl

Preparation Time: 20 minutes
Cooking Time: 25 minutes
Yield: 2 servings

Ingredients:

- 2 medium sweet potatoes, peeled and diced
- 1 can (15 oz) chickpeas, drained and rinsed
- 2 tablespoons olive oil
- 1 teaspoon smoked paprika
- 1 teaspoon ground cumin
- 1 teaspoon garlic powder
- Salt and black pepper to taste
- 2 cups cooked quinoa
- 2 cups mixed greens
- 1 avocado, sliced
- Tahini dressing for drizzling

Procedure:

1. **Roast Sweet Potatoes and Chickpeas:**
   - Preheat the oven to 425°F (220°C). Toss diced sweet potatoes and chickpeas with olive oil, smoked paprika, cumin, garlic powder, salt, and black pepper. Roast for 25 minutes or until golden and crispy.
2. **Assemble Bowls:**
   - Divide cooked quinoa, mixed greens, roasted sweet potatoes, and chickpeas into bowls.
3. **Add Avocado:**
   - Top each bowl with sliced avocado.
4. **Drizzle with Tahini Dressing:**
   - Drizzle tahini dressing over the Buddha bowls.
5. **Serve:**
   - Serve immediately as a wholesome Sweet Potato and Chickpea Buddha Bowl.

Vegetable and Brown Rice Sushi Rolls

Preparation Time: 30 minutes
Yield: 4 servings

Ingredients:

- 2 cups brown rice, cooked and seasoned with rice vinegar
- 4 sheets nori (seaweed)
- 1 cucumber, julienned
- 1 carrot, julienned
- 1 avocado, sliced
- 1/2 cup pickled ginger
- Low-sodium soy sauce for dipping
- Wasabi and sesame seeds for garnish

Procedure:

1. **Prepare Sushi Rice:**
   - Cook brown rice according to package instructions. Season with rice vinegar.
2. **Place Nori Sheets:**
   - Lay a bamboo sushi rolling mat on a flat surface. Place a sheet of nori on the mat.
3. **Spread Rice on Nori:**
   - Wet your hands and spread a thin layer of seasoned brown rice evenly over the nori, leaving a small border at the top.
4. **Add Vegetables:**
   - Arrange julienned cucumber, julienned carrot, and avocado slices in the center of the rice.
5. **Roll Sushi:**
   - Carefully roll the sushi using the bamboo mat, applying gentle pressure. Seal the edge with a bit of water.
6. **Slice Rolls:**
   - Using a sharp knife, slice the sushi roll into bite-sized pieces.
7. **Serve:**

- Serve Vegetable and Brown Rice Sushi Rolls with pickled ginger, soy sauce, wasabi, and a sprinkle of sesame seeds.

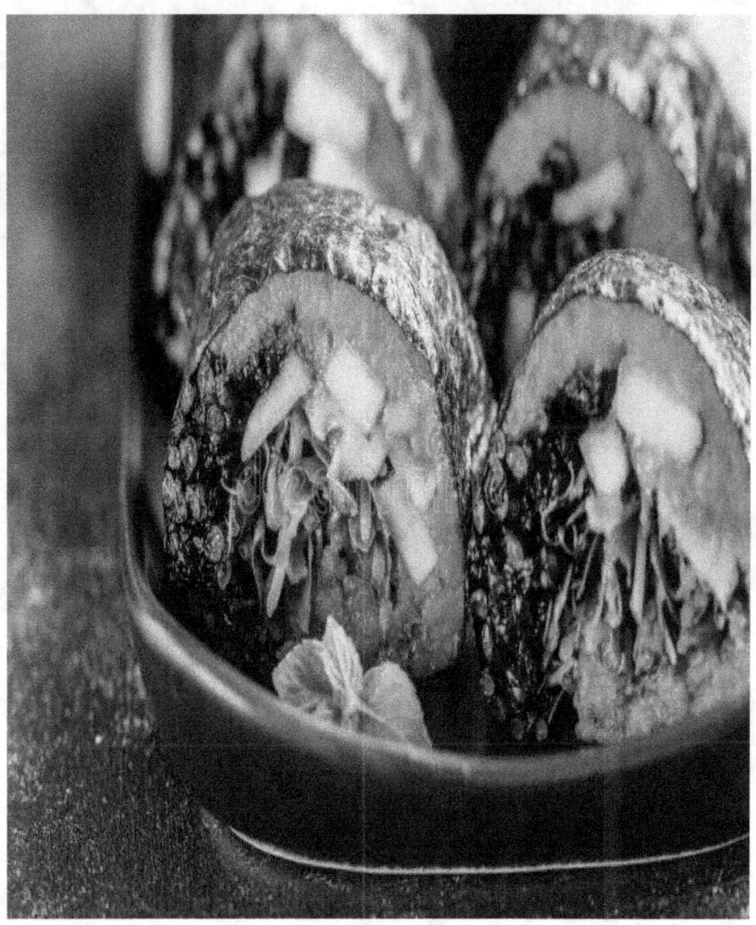

Grilled Portobello Mushroom Sandwich

Preparation Time: 15 minutes
Cooking Time: 10 minutes
Yield: 2 servings

Ingredients:

- 4 large Portobello mushroom caps
- 2 tablespoons balsamic vinegar
- 2 tablespoons olive oil
- 2 cloves garlic, minced
- Salt and black pepper to taste
- 4 whole grain buns
- 1 cup arugula
- 1 tomato, sliced
- 1/2 cup goat cheese, crumbled

Procedure:

1. **Marinate Mushrooms:**
   - In a bowl, whisk together balsamic vinegar, olive oil, minced garlic, salt, and black pepper. Brush the mushroom caps with the marinade.
2. **Grill Mushrooms:**
   - Preheat the grill or grill pan. Grill the marinated mushroom caps for 4-5 minutes per side, or until tender.
3. **Prepare Buns:**
   - Toast the whole grain buns on the grill.
4. **Assemble Sandwiches:**
   - Place grilled portobello mushrooms on the toasted buns. Top with arugula, sliced tomato, and crumbled goat cheese.
5. **Serve:**
   - Serve Grilled Portobello Mushroom Sandwiches immediately.

Zucchini Noodles with Pesto and Cherry Tomatoes

Preparation Time: 15 minutes
Cooking Time: 5 minutes
Yield: 2 servings

Ingredients:

- 2 large zucchini, spiralized into noodles
- 1 cup cherry tomatoes, halved
- 1/3 cup pesto sauce
- 1/4 cup pine nuts, toasted
- Grated Parmesan cheese for garnish
- Fresh basil leaves for garnish

Procedure:

1. **Prepare Zucchini Noodles:**
   - Spiralize zucchini into noodles using a spiralizer.
2. **Sauté Noodles:**
   - In a large skillet, sauté zucchini noodles over medium heat for 3-5 minutes until just tender.
3. **Add Cherry Tomatoes:**
   - Add halved cherry tomatoes to the skillet and cook for an additional 2 minutes.
4. **Toss with Pesto:**
   - Stir in pesto sauce, ensuring the noodles and tomatoes are well coated.
5. **Toast Pine Nuts:**
   - In a separate pan, toast pine nuts until golden.
6. **Serve:**
   - Divide Zucchini Noodles with Pesto and Cherry Tomatoes into plates. Garnish with toasted pine nuts, grated Parmesan cheese, and fresh basil leaves.

Quinoa Salad with Roasted Vegetables

Preparation Time: 20 minutes
Cooking Time: 25 minutes
Yield: 4 servings

Ingredients:

- 1 cup quinoa, rinsed
- 2 cups mixed vegetables (e.g., bell peppers, zucchini, cherry tomatoes), chopped
- 2 tablespoons olive oil
- 1 teaspoon dried thyme
- 1 teaspoon dried rosemary
- Salt and black pepper to taste
- 1/4 cup feta cheese, crumbled
- 2 tablespoons balsamic vinaigrette

Procedure:

1. **Cook Quinoa:**
   - Cook quinoa according to package instructions.
2. **Roast Vegetables:**
   - Preheat the oven to 425°F (220°C). Toss chopped vegetables with olive oil, dried thyme, dried rosemary, salt, and black pepper. Roast for 20-25 minutes or until vegetables are tender.
3. **Assemble Salad:**
   - In a large bowl, combine cooked quinoa, roasted vegetables, crumbled feta cheese, and balsamic vinaigrette. Toss gently to mix.
4. **Serve:**
   - Serve Quinoa Salad with Roasted Vegetables as a delightful and nutritious dish.

Teriyaki Tofu Stir-Fry

Preparation Time: 20 minutes
Cooking Time: 10 minutes
Yield: 2 servings

Ingredients:

- 1 block firm tofu, pressed and cubed
- 2 cups broccoli florets
- 1 bell pepper, sliced
- 1 carrot, julienned
- 2 tablespoons low-sodium teriyaki sauce
- 1 tablespoon soy sauce
- 1 tablespoon sesame oil
- 1 teaspoon ginger, minced
- 2 cloves garlic, minced
- 1 tablespoon sesame seeds
- Green onions for garnish

Procedure:

1. **Press Tofu:**
   - Press firm tofu to remove excess water, then cut into cubes.
2. **Stir-Fry Tofu:**
   - In a large skillet or wok, heat sesame oil over medium-high heat. Add cubed tofu and cook until golden on all sides.
3. **Add Vegetables:**
   - Add broccoli, bell pepper, carrot, minced ginger, and minced garlic to the skillet. Stir-fry until vegetables are tender-crisp.
4. **Pour Sauces:**
   - Pour low-sodium teriyaki sauce and soy sauce over the tofu and vegetables. Toss to coat evenly.
5. **Garnish and Serve:**

- Sprinkle sesame seeds and garnish with sliced green onions. Serve the Teriyaki Tofu Stir-Fry over brown rice or quinoa

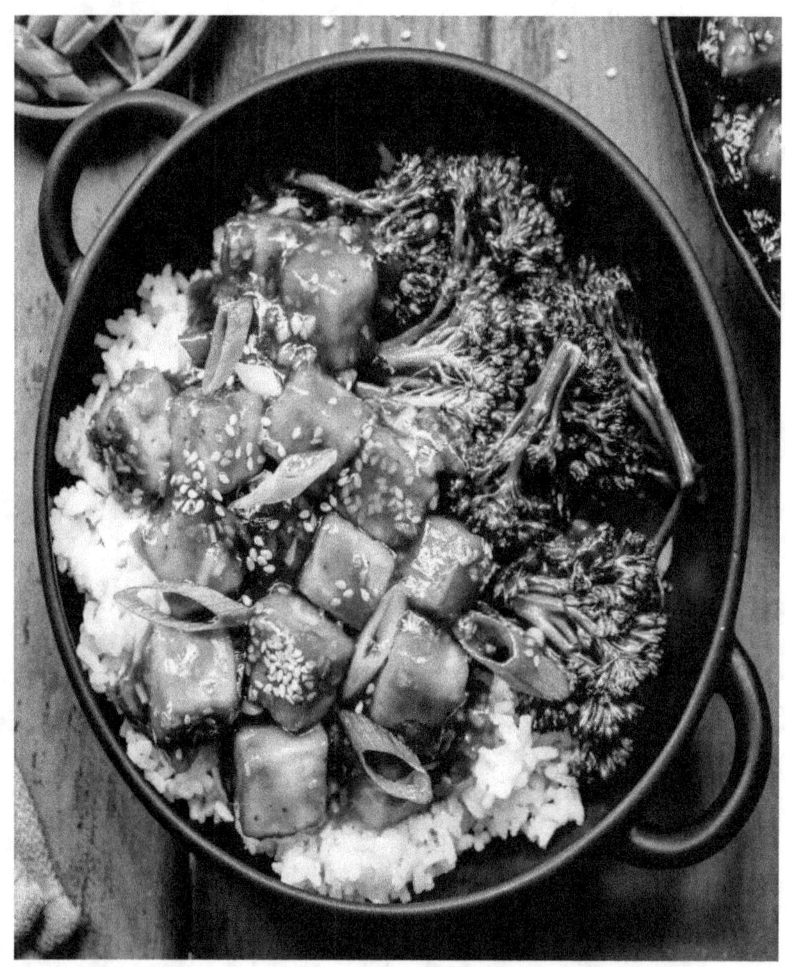

Eggplant and Chickpea Stew

Preparation Time: 15 minutes
Cooking Time: 30 minutes
Yield: 4 servings

Ingredients:

- 1 large eggplant, diced
- 1 can (15 oz) chickpeas, drained and rinsed
- 1 onion, diced
- 2 bell peppers, diced
- 3 cloves garlic, minced
- 1 can (15 oz) diced tomatoes
- 1 teaspoon ground cumin
- 1 teaspoon smoked paprika
- 1/2 teaspoon chili powder
- Salt and black pepper to taste
- Fresh parsley for garnish

Procedure:

1. **Saute Vegetables:**
   - In a large pot, sauté diced eggplant, diced onion, diced bell peppers, and minced garlic until vegetables are softened.
2. **Add Chickpeas and Tomatoes:**
   - Add chickpeas and diced tomatoes (with their juice) to the pot. Stir to combine.
3. **Season and Simmer:**
   - Season with ground cumin, smoked paprika, chili powder, salt, and black pepper. Simmer for 25-30 minutes until the stew thickens.
4. **Adjust Seasoning:**
   - Taste and adjust seasoning as needed.
5. **Garnish and Serve:**
   - Garnish with fresh parsley and serve the Eggplant and Chickpea Stew over quinoa or couscous.

Black Bean and Quinoa Stuffed Bell Peppers

Preparation Time: 25 minutes
Cooking Time: 30 minutes
Yield: 4 servings

Ingredients:

- 4 large bell peppers, halved and seeds removed
- 1 cup cooked quinoa
- 1 can (15 oz) black beans, drained and rinsed
- 1 cup corn kernels (fresh or frozen)
- 1 cup cherry tomatoes, diced
- 1/2 cup red onion, finely chopped
- 1 teaspoon cumin
- 1 teaspoon chili powder
- Salt and pepper to taste
- 1 cup shredded low-fat cheddar cheese

Procedure:

1. **Preheat Oven:**
   - Preheat the oven to 375°F (190°C).
2. **Prepare Peppers:**
   - Place bell pepper halves in a baking dish.
3. **Mix Filling:**
   - In a bowl, combine cooked quinoa, black beans, cherry tomatoes, corn, red onion, cumin, chili powder, salt, and pepper.
4. **Stuff Peppers:**
   - Fill each bell pepper half with the quinoa and vegetable mixture.
5. **Top with Cheese:**
   - Sprinkle shredded cheddar cheese over the stuffed peppers.
6. **Bake:**
   - Bake in the preheated oven for 25-30 minutes or until the peppers are tender and the cheese is melted and bubbly.

7. **Serve:**
   - Serve Black Bean and Quinoa Stuffed Bell Peppers hot, garnished with fresh cilantro if desired

Lentil and Vegetable Curry

Preparation Time: 20 minutes
Cooking Time: 30 minutes
Yield: 4 servings

Ingredients:

- 1 cup dry lentils, rinsed
- 3 cups vegetable broth
- 1 onion, diced
- 2 carrots, diced
- 1 bell pepper, diced
- 2 cups cauliflower florets
- 3 cloves garlic, minced
- 1 tablespoon curry powder
- 1 teaspoon ground cumin
- 1 teaspoon ground coriander
- 1 can (14 oz) coconut milk
- Salt and black pepper to taste
- Fresh cilantro for garnish

Procedure:

1. **Cook Lentils:**
   - In a pot, combine dry lentils and vegetable broth. Bring to a boil, then reduce heat and simmer for 15-20 minutes or until lentils are tender.
2. **Sauté Vegetables:**

- In a large skillet, sauté diced onion, diced carrots, diced bell pepper, cauliflower florets, and minced garlic until vegetables are softened.

3. **Add Spices:**
   - Stir in curry powder, ground cumin, and ground coriander. Cook for an additional 2 minutes.

4. **Combine Lentils and Vegetables:**
   - Add cooked lentils and coconut milk to the skillet. Stir to combine. Simmer for 10 minutes.

5. **Season and Garnish:**
   - Season with salt and black pepper. Garnish with fresh cilantro before serving.

6. **Serve:**
   - Serve Lentil and Vegetable Curry over brown rice or quinoa.

Dinner Wonders

Grilled Salmon with Lemon-Dill Sauce

Preparation Time: 10 minutes
Cooking Time: 10 minutes
Yield: 2 servings

Ingredients:

- 2 salmon fillets
- 1 tablespoon olive oil
- 1 teaspoon lemon zest
- 2 tablespoons lemon juice
- 1 tablespoon fresh dill, chopped
- Salt and black pepper to taste

Procedure:

1. **Preheat Grill:**
   - Preheat the grill to medium-high heat.
2. **Prepare Salmon:**
   - Brush salmon fillets with olive oil and season with salt and black pepper.
3. **Grill Salmon:**
   - Grill salmon for 4-5 minutes per side, or until it flakes easily with a fork.
4. **Make Lemon-Dill Sauce:**
   - In a small bowl, mix lemon zest, lemon juice, and chopped dill to create the sauce.
5. **Serve:**
   - Drizzle the grilled salmon with the lemon-dill sauce and serve immediately.

Quinoa-Stuffed Bell Peppers

Preparation Time: 20 minutes
Cooking Time: 30 minutes
Yield: 4 servings

Ingredients:

- 4 large bell peppers, halved and seeds removed
- 1 cup cooked quinoa
- 1 can (15 oz) black beans, drained and rinsed
- 1 cup corn kernels (fresh or frozen)
- 1 cup cherry tomatoes, diced
- 1/2 cup red onion, finely chopped
- 1 teaspoon cumin
- 1 teaspoon chili powder
- Salt and pepper to taste
- 1 cup shredded low-fat cheddar cheese

Procedure:

1. **Preheat Oven:**
   - Preheat the oven to 375°F (190°C).
2. **Prepare Peppers:**
   - Place bell pepper halves in a baking dish.
3. **Mix Filling:**
   - In a bowl, combine cooked quinoa, black beans, cherry tomatoes, corn, red onion, cumin, chili powder, salt, and pepper.
4. **Stuff Peppers:**
   - Fill each bell pepper half with the quinoa and vegetable mixture.
5. **Top with Cheese:**
   - Sprinkle shredded cheddar cheese over the stuffed peppers.
6. **Bake:**
   - Bake in the preheated oven for 25-30 minutes or until the peppers are tender and the cheese is melted and bubbly.

7. **Serve:**
   - Serve Quinoa-Stuffed Bell Peppers hot, garnished with fresh cilantro if desired.

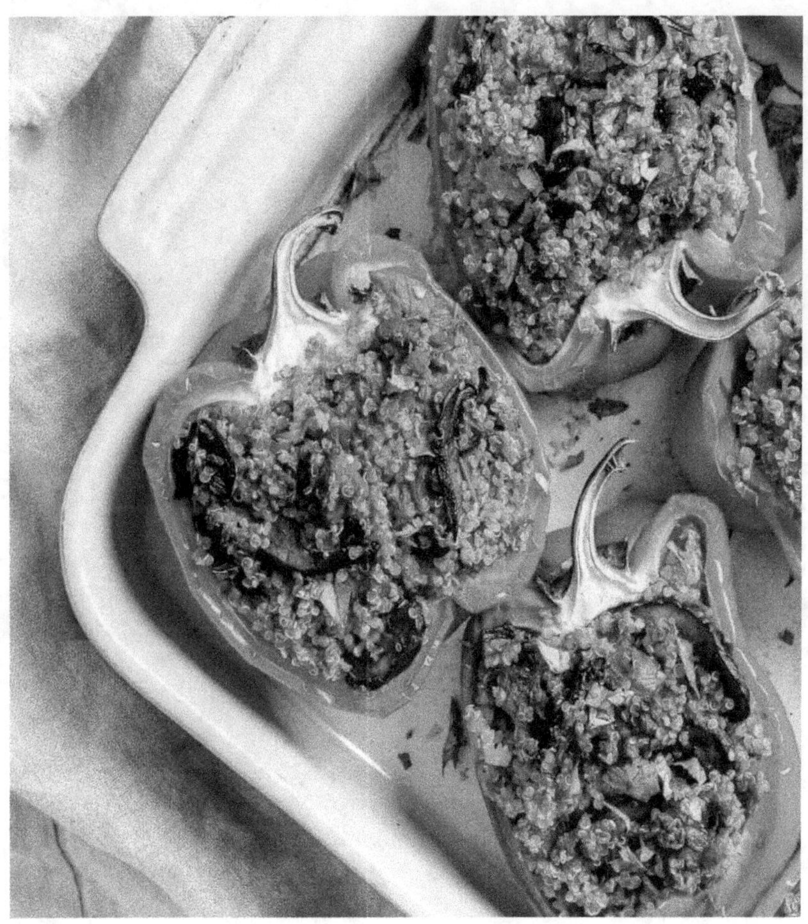

Baked Chicken Breast with Herbs

Preparation Time: 15 minutes
Cooking Time: 25 minutes
Yield: 2 servings

Ingredients:

- 2 boneless, skinless chicken breasts
- 2 tablespoons olive oil
- 1 teaspoon dried thyme
- 1 teaspoon dried rosemary
- 1 teaspoon garlic powder
- Salt and black pepper to taste
- Fresh lemon wedges for serving

Procedure:

1. **Preheat Oven:**
   - Preheat the oven to 400°F (200°C).
2. **Prepare Chicken:**
   - Rub chicken breasts with olive oil, dried thyme, dried rosemary, garlic powder, salt, and black pepper.
3. **Bake Chicken:**
   - Place chicken on a baking sheet and bake for 20-25 minutes or until the internal temperature reaches 165°F (74°C).
4. **Rest:**
   - Let the chicken rest for a few minutes before slicing.
5. **Serve:**
   - Serve Baked Chicken Breast with Herbs with fresh lemon wedges on the side.

Lentil and Vegetable Stir-Fry

Preparation Time: 20 minutes
Cooking Time: 15 minutes
Yield: 4 servings

Ingredients:

- 1 cup dry lentils, rinsed
- 3 cups vegetable broth
- 2 tablespoons soy sauce
- 1 tablespoon sesame oil
- 1 tablespoon rice vinegar
- 1 tablespoon ginger, minced
- 2 cloves garlic, minced
- 2 cups broccoli florets
- 1 red bell pepper, sliced
- 1 carrot, julienned
- 1 cup snap peas, trimmed
- Green onions for garnish
- Sesame seeds for garnish

Procedure:

1. **Cook Lentils:**
   - In a pot, combine dry lentils and vegetable broth. Bring to a boil, then reduce heat and simmer for 15-20 minutes or until lentils are tender.
2. **Prepare Sauce:**
   - In a small bowl, mix soy sauce, sesame oil, rice vinegar, minced ginger, and minced garlic to create the sauce.
3. **Stir-Fry Vegetables:**
   - In a wok or large skillet, stir-fry broccoli, red bell pepper, julienned carrot, and snap peas until crisp-tender.
4. **Add Lentils and Sauce:**
   - Add cooked lentils to the stir-fried vegetables. Pour the sauce over the mixture and toss to coat evenly.
5. **Garnish and Serve:**

- Garnish with chopped green onions and sesame seeds. Serve Lentil and Vegetable Stir-Fry over brown rice or quinoa.

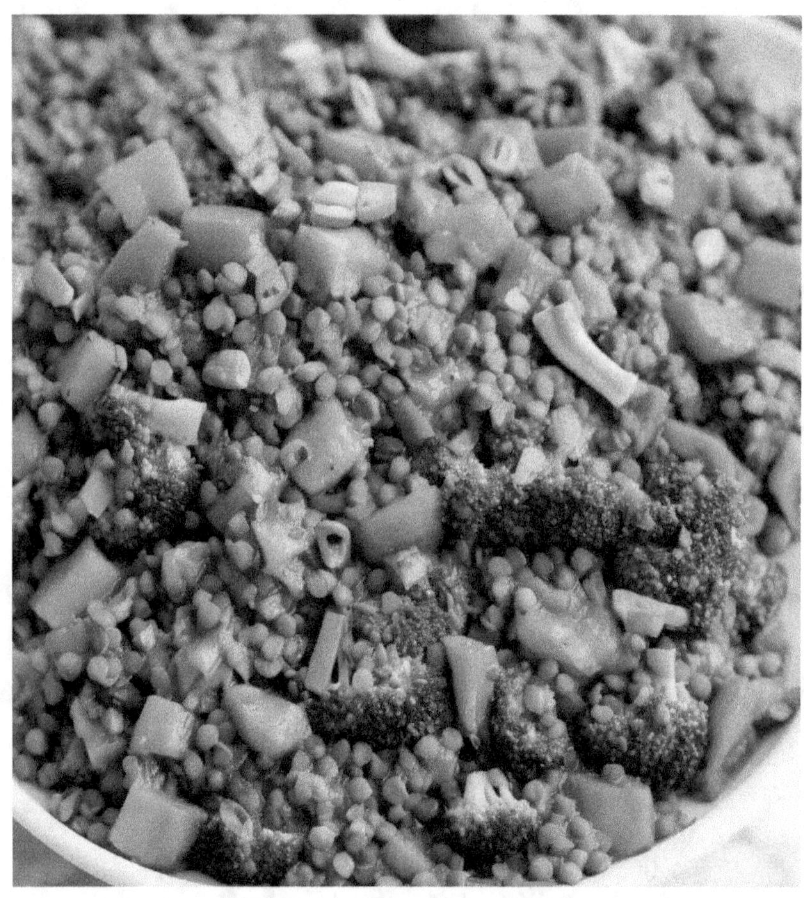

Shrimp and Asparagus Skewers

Preparation Time: 15 minutes
Cooking Time: 10 minutes
Yield: 2 servings

Ingredients:

- 1/2 pound large shrimp, peeled and deveined
- 1 bunch asparagus, trimmed
- 2 tablespoons olive oil
- 1 teaspoon lemon zest
- 2 tablespoons lemon juice
- 1 teaspoon garlic, minced
- Salt and black pepper to taste
- Wooden skewers, soaked in water

Procedure:

1. **Preheat Grill:**
   - Preheat the grill to medium-high heat.
2. **Prepare Skewers:**
   - Thread shrimp and asparagus onto wooden skewers, alternating between them.
3. **Make Marinade:**
   - In a bowl, whisk together olive oil, lemon zest, lemon juice, minced garlic, salt, and black pepper to create the marinade.
4. **Grill Skewers:**
   - Grill skewers for 2-3 minutes per side, or until shrimp are opaque and asparagus is tender.
5. **Serve:**
   - Drizzle the skewers with any remaining marinade and serve Shrimp and Asparagus Skewers immediately.

Mediterranean Chickpea Salad

Preparation Time: 15 minutes
Yield: 4 servings

Ingredients:

- 2 cans (15 oz each) chickpeas, drained and rinsed
- 1 cucumber, diced
- 1 cup cherry tomatoes, halved
- 1/2 red onion, finely chopped
- 1/2 cup Kalamata olives, sliced
- 1/2 cup feta cheese, crumbled
- 1/4 cup fresh parsley, chopped
- 3 tablespoons olive oil
- 2 tablespoons red wine vinegar
- Salt and black pepper to taste

Procedure:

1. **Combine *Ingredients*:**
   - In a large bowl, combine chickpeas, diced cucumber, cherry tomatoes, finely chopped red onion, sliced Kalamata olives, crumbled feta cheese, and chopped fresh parsley.
2. **Make Dressing:**
   - In a small bowl, whisk together olive oil, red wine vinegar, salt, and black pepper to create the dressing.
3. **Toss and Coat:**
   - Pour the dressing over the chickpea mixture. Toss gently to coat everything evenly.
4. **Chill:**
   - Chill the Mediterranean Chickpea Salad in the refrigerator for at least 30 minutes before serving.
5. **Serve:**
   - Serve chilled, and adjust salt and pepper to taste if needed.

Spaghetti Squash Primavera

Preparation Time: 15 minutes
Cooking Time: 40 minutes
Yield: 4 servings

Ingredients:

- 1 large spaghetti squash, halved and seeds removed
- 2 tablespoons olive oil
- 1 onion, diced
- 2 bell peppers (assorted colors), sliced
- 2 carrots, julienned
- 2 zucchinis, diced
- 2 cloves garlic, minced
- 1 can (14 oz) diced tomatoes, drained
- 1 teaspoon dried oregano
- 1 teaspoon dried basil
- Salt and black pepper to taste
- Grated Parmesan cheese for garnish (optional)

Procedure:

1. **Preheat Oven:**
   - Preheat the oven to 400°F (200°C).
2. **Roast Spaghetti Squash:**
   - Place spaghetti squash halves on a baking sheet, cut side down. Roast for 30-40 minutes or until the squash is fork-tender.
3. **Prepare Vegetables:**
   - While the squash is roasting, heat olive oil in a large skillet. Add diced onion, sliced bell peppers, julienned carrots, diced zucchinis, and minced garlic. Sauté until vegetables are tender-crisp.
4. **Scrape Squash Strands:**
   - Once the spaghetti squash is cooked, use a fork to scrape the strands from the skin.
5. **Combine and Season:**

- Add the spaghetti squash strands to the skillet with
  sautéed vegetables. Add drained diced tomatoes, dried
  oregano, dried basil, salt, and black pepper. Toss
  everything together.

6. **Garnish and Serve:**
   - Garnish with grated Parmesan cheese if desired. Serve
     Spaghetti Squash Primavera warm.

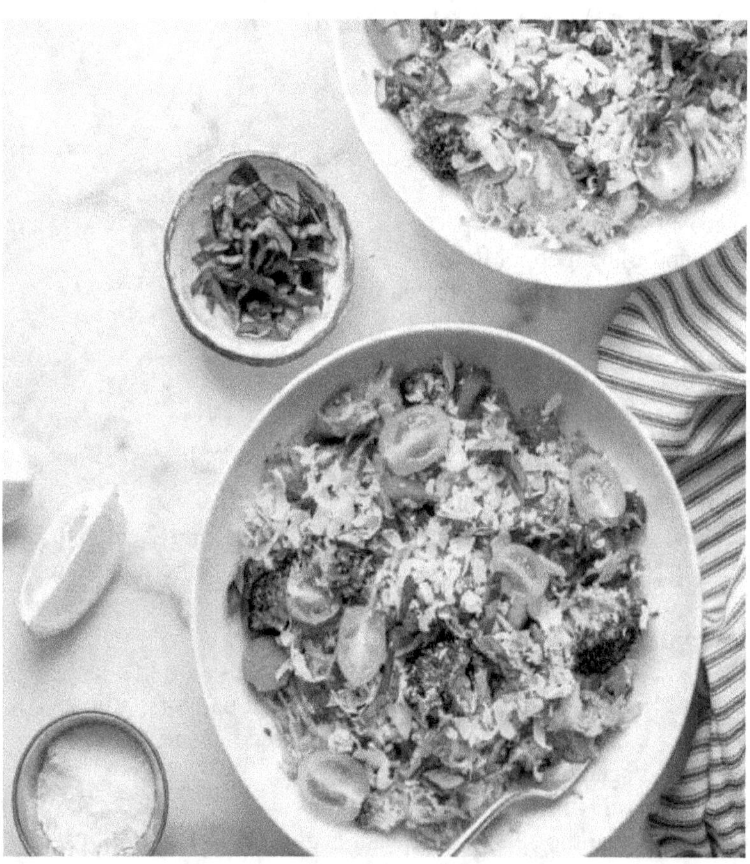

Teriyaki Tofu and Vegetable Skewers

Preparation Time: 20 minutes
Cooking Time: 10 minutes
Yield: 4 servings

Ingredients:

- 1 block firm tofu, pressed and cubed
- 2 cups broccoli florets
- 1 bell pepper, sliced
- 1 zucchini, sliced
- 1/2 cup teriyaki sauce
- 2 tablespoons soy sauce
- 1 tablespoon sesame oil
- 1 teaspoon ginger, minced
- 2 cloves garlic, minced
- Wooden skewers, soaked in water

Procedure:

1. **Press Tofu:**
   - Press firm tofu to remove excess water, then cut into cubes.
2. **Prepare Marinade:**
   - In a bowl, whisk together teriyaki sauce, soy sauce, sesame oil, minced ginger, and minced garlic.
3. **Marinate Tofu:**
   - Place tofu cubes in a shallow dish and pour half of the marinade over them. Let it marinate for at least 15 minutes.
4. **Assemble Skewers:**
   - Thread marinated tofu cubes, broccoli florets, sliced bell pepper, and sliced zucchini onto wooden skewers, alternating between them.
5. **Grill Skewers:**
   - Grill skewers for 4-5 minutes per side or until the tofu is golden and vegetables are tender.
6. **Brush with Marinade:**

- While grilling, brush the skewers with the remaining marinade for added flavor.

7. **Serve:**
   - Serve Teriyaki Tofu and Vegetable Skewers hot, and drizzle with any remaining marinade.

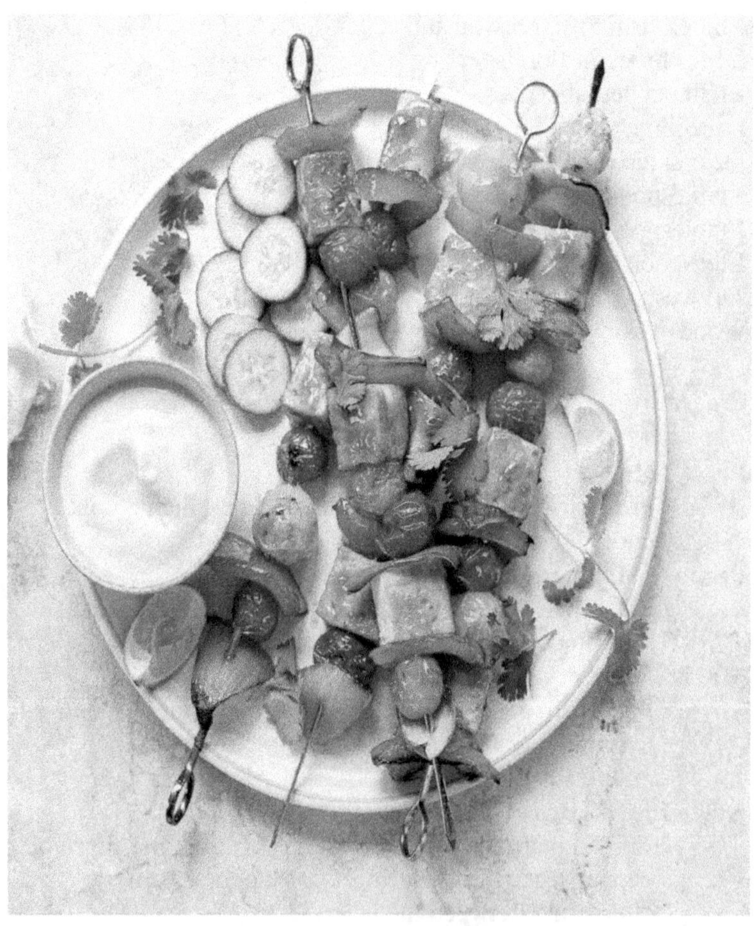

Lemon Garlic Roasted Chicken Thighs

Preparation Time: 10 minutes
Cooking Time: 35 minutes
Yield: 4 servings

Ingredients:

- 8 bone-in, skin-on chicken thighs
- 3 tablespoons olive oil
- 4 cloves garlic, minced
- 1 teaspoon lemon zest
- 2 tablespoons lemon juice
- 1 teaspoon dried thyme
- 1 teaspoon dried rosemary
- Salt and black pepper to taste
- Fresh parsley for garnish

Procedure:

1. **Preheat Oven:**
   - Preheat the oven to 400°F (200°C).
2. **Prepare Chicken Thighs:**
   - Pat chicken thighs dry with paper towels. Place them in a large bowl.
3. **Make Marinade:**
   - In a small bowl, whisk together olive oil, minced garlic, lemon zest, lemon juice, dried thyme, dried rosemary, salt, and black pepper.
4. **Marinate Chicken:**
   - Pour the marinade over the chicken thighs. Toss to coat evenly and let them marinate for at least 10 minutes.
5. **Roast Chicken:**
   - Place the chicken thighs on a baking sheet, skin side up. Roast in the preheated oven for 30-35 minutes or until the internal temperature reaches 165°F (74°C) and the skin is crispy.
6. **Garnish and Serve:**

- Garnish with fresh parsley and serve Lemon Garlic Roasted Chicken Thighs hot.

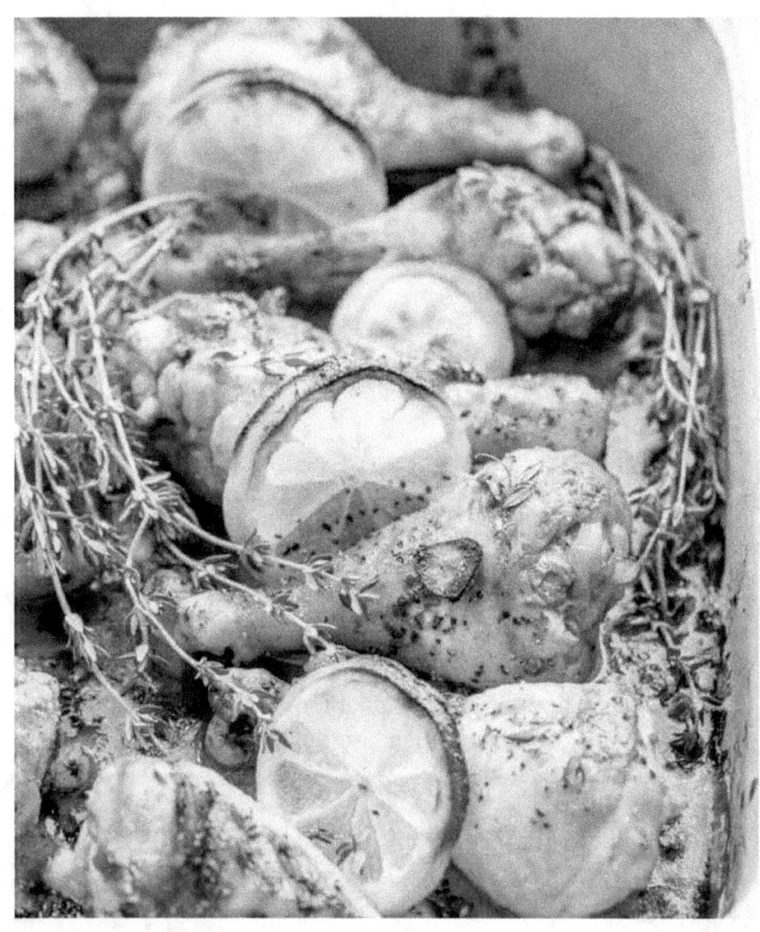

Eggplant Parmesan

Preparation Time: 30 minutes
Cooking Time: 40 minutes
Yield: 4 servings

Ingredients:

- 2 large eggplants, sliced into rounds
- 2 cups whole wheat breadcrumbs
- 1 cup grated Parmesan cheese
- 3 eggs, beaten
- 2 cups marinara sauce
- 2 cups part-skim mozzarella cheese, shredded
- Fresh basil for garnish

Procedure:

1. **Preheat Oven:**
   - Preheat the oven to 375°F (190°C).
2. **Coat Eggplant Slices:**
   - Dip eggplant slices into beaten eggs, then coat with a mixture of whole wheat breadcrumbs and grated Parmesan cheese.
3. **Bake Eggplant:**
   - Place coated eggplant slices on a baking sheet and bake for 20 minutes, or until golden brown and crispy.
4. **Layer with Sauce and Cheese:**
   - In a baking dish, layer half of the baked eggplant slices. Top with marinara sauce and shredded mozzarella cheese. Repeat the layers.
5. **Bake Until Bubbly:**
   - Bake in the preheated oven for an additional 20 minutes or until the cheese is melted and bubbly.
6. **Garnish and Serve:**
   - Garnish Eggplant Parmesan with fresh basil and serve warm.

Butternut Squash and Black Bean Chili

Preparation Time: 20 minutes
Cooking Time: 30 minutes
Yield: 4 servings

Ingredients:

- 2 cups butternut squash, diced
- 1 can (15 oz) black beans, drained and rinsed
- 1 can (14 oz) diced tomatoes, untrained
- 1 onion, diced
- 2 cloves garlic, minced
- 1 bell pepper, diced
- 1 tablespoon chili powder
- 1 teaspoon cumin
- 1 teaspoon paprika
- 1/2 teaspoon cinnamon
- Salt and black pepper to taste
- Fresh cilantro for garnish

Procedure:

1. **Sauté Vegetables:**
   - In a large pot, sauté diced butternut squash, diced onion, minced garlic, and diced bell pepper until vegetables are softened.
2. **Add Seasonings:**
   - Stir in chili powder, cumin, paprika, cinnamon, salt, and black pepper. Cook for an additional 2 minutes.
3. **Combine *Ingredients*:**
   - Add drained black beans and undrained diced tomatoes to the pot. Stir to combine.
4. **Simmer:**
   - Simmer the chili over medium heat for 20-25 minutes or until the butternut squash is tender.
5. **Adjust Seasoning and Serve:**

- Adjust seasoning if necessary. Garnish with fresh cilantro and serve Butternut Squash and Black Bean Chili hot.

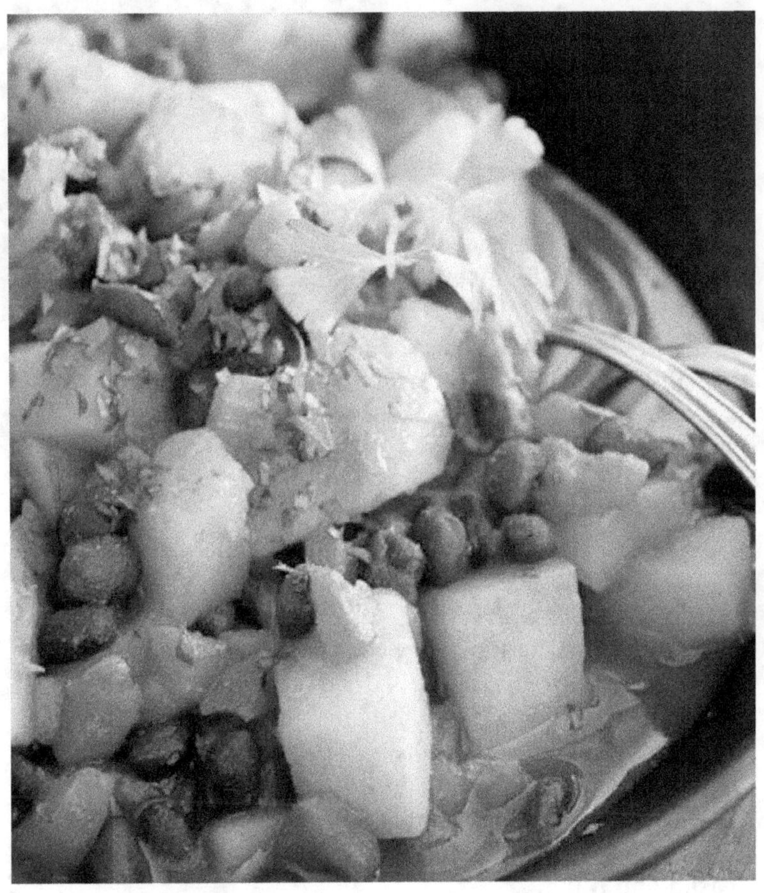

Spinach and Feta Stuffed Chicken Breast

Preparation Time: 20 minutes
Cooking Time: 25 minutes
Yield: 4 servings

Ingredients:

- 4 boneless, skinless chicken breasts
- 2 cups fresh spinach, chopped
- 1/2 cup feta cheese, crumbled
- 2 cloves garlic, minced
- 1 tablespoon olive oil
- 1 teaspoon dried oregano
- 1 teaspoon dried thyme
- Salt and black pepper to taste
- Lemon wedges for serving

Procedure:

1. **Preheat Oven:**
   - Preheat the oven to 400°F (200°C).
2. **Butterfly Chicken Breasts:**
   - Butterfly each chicken breast by making a horizontal cut along the side, without cutting all the way through.
3. **Sauté Spinach Mixture:**
   - In a skillet, sauté chopped spinach, crumbled feta cheese, minced garlic, olive oil, dried oregano, and dried thyme until the spinach wilts and the mixture is well combined.
4. **Stuff Chicken Breasts:**
   - Open the butterflied chicken breasts and evenly divide the spinach and feta mixture among them. Close the chicken breasts and secure with toothpicks if needed.
5. **Season and Bake:**
   - Season the stuffed chicken breasts with salt and black pepper. Place them on a baking sheet and bake for 20-25 minutes or until the internal temperature reaches 165°F (74°C).
6. **Rest and Serve:**

- Let the stuffed chicken breasts rest for a few minutes before slicing. Serve with lemon wedges.

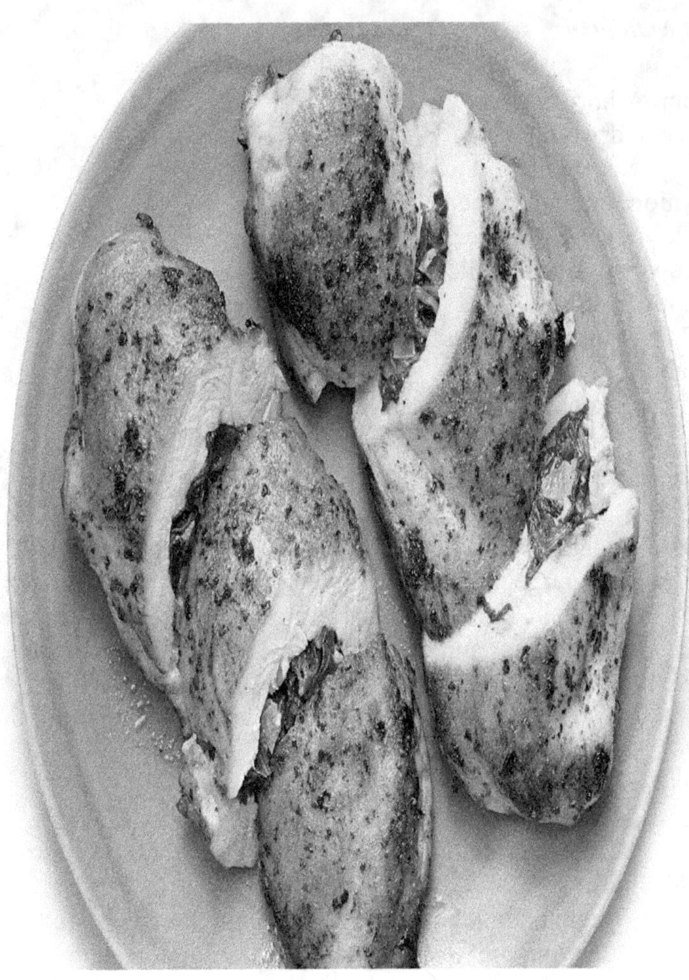

Mushroom and Spinach Risotto

Preparation Time: 15 minutes
Cooking Time: 30 minutes
Yield: 4 servings

Ingredients:

- 1 cup Arborio rice
- 1/2 cup dry white wine
- 4 cups vegetable broth, heated
- 1 onion, finely chopped
- 2 cloves garlic, minced
- 2 cups mushrooms, sliced
- 2 cups fresh spinach
- 1/2 cup Parmesan cheese, grated
- 2 tablespoons butter
- Salt and black pepper to taste

Procedure:

1. **Sauté Vegetables:**
   - In a large pan, sauté finely chopped onion and minced garlic in 1 tablespoon of butter until softened. Add sliced mushrooms and cook until they release their moisture.
2. **Toast Rice:**
   - Add Arborio rice to the pan and cook, stirring, until the rice is lightly toasted.
3. **Deglaze with Wine:**
   - Pour in dry white wine to deglaze the pan, stirring constantly until the wine is absorbed.
4. **Add Broth:**
   - Begin adding heated vegetable broth, one ladle at a time, allowing the rice to absorb the liquid before adding more. Stir continuously.
5. **Finish with Spinach and Cheese:**
   - When the rice is almost tender, stir in fresh spinach, grated Parmesan cheese, and the remaining butter.

Continue to cook until the spinach wilts and the cheese melts.

6. **Adjust Seasoning and Serve:**
    - Season with salt and black pepper to taste. Risotto is ready when it reaches a creamy consistency. Serve Mushroom and Spinach Risotto hot.

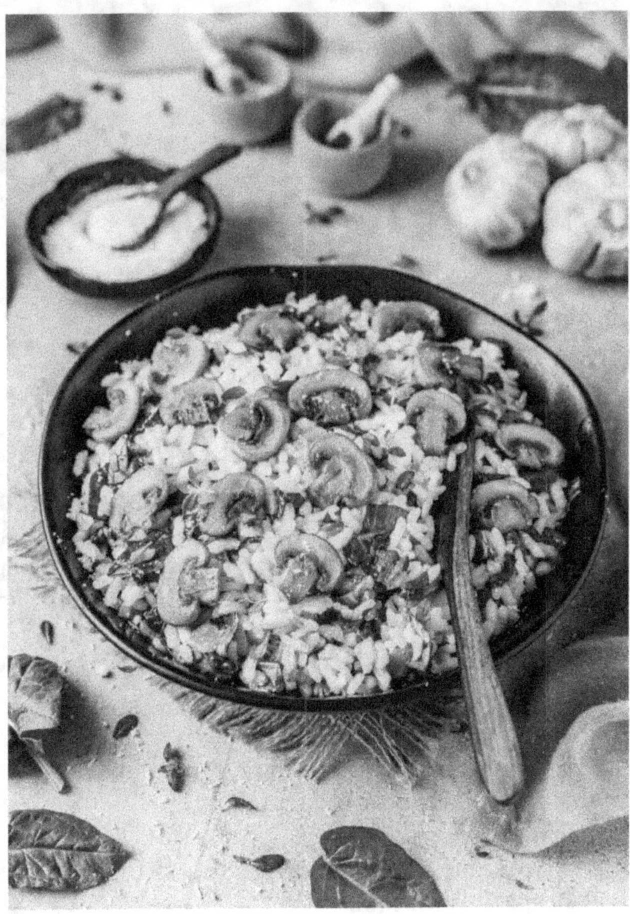

Turkey and Vegetable Meatballs

Preparation Time: 20 minutes
Cooking Time: 20 minutes
Yield: 4 servings

Ingredients:

- 1 pound lean ground turkey
- 1/2 cup whole wheat breadcrumbs
- 1/4 cup grated Parmesan cheese
- 1/4 cup fresh parsley, chopped
- 1 egg, beaten
- 2 cloves garlic, minced
- 1 teaspoon dried oregano
- 1 teaspoon dried basil
- Salt and black pepper to taste
- 2 cups marinara sauce

Procedure:

1. **Preheat Oven:**
   - Preheat the oven to 375°F (190°C).
2. **Mix Meatball *Ingredients*:**
   - In a bowl, combine ground turkey, whole wheat breadcrumbs, grated Parmesan cheese, chopped fresh parsley, beaten egg, minced garlic, dried oregano, dried basil, salt, and black pepper. Mix until well combined.
3. **Form Meatballs:**
   - Shape the mixture into meatballs of equal size and place them on a baking sheet.
4. **Bake:**
   - Bake in the preheated oven for 18-20 minutes or until the meatballs are cooked through.
5. **Warm Marinara Sauce:**
   - While the meatballs are baking, heat marinara sauce in a saucepan over medium heat.
6. **Serve:**

- Once the meatballs are done, serve them with warm marinara sauce. Enjoy Turkey and Vegetable Meatballs hot.

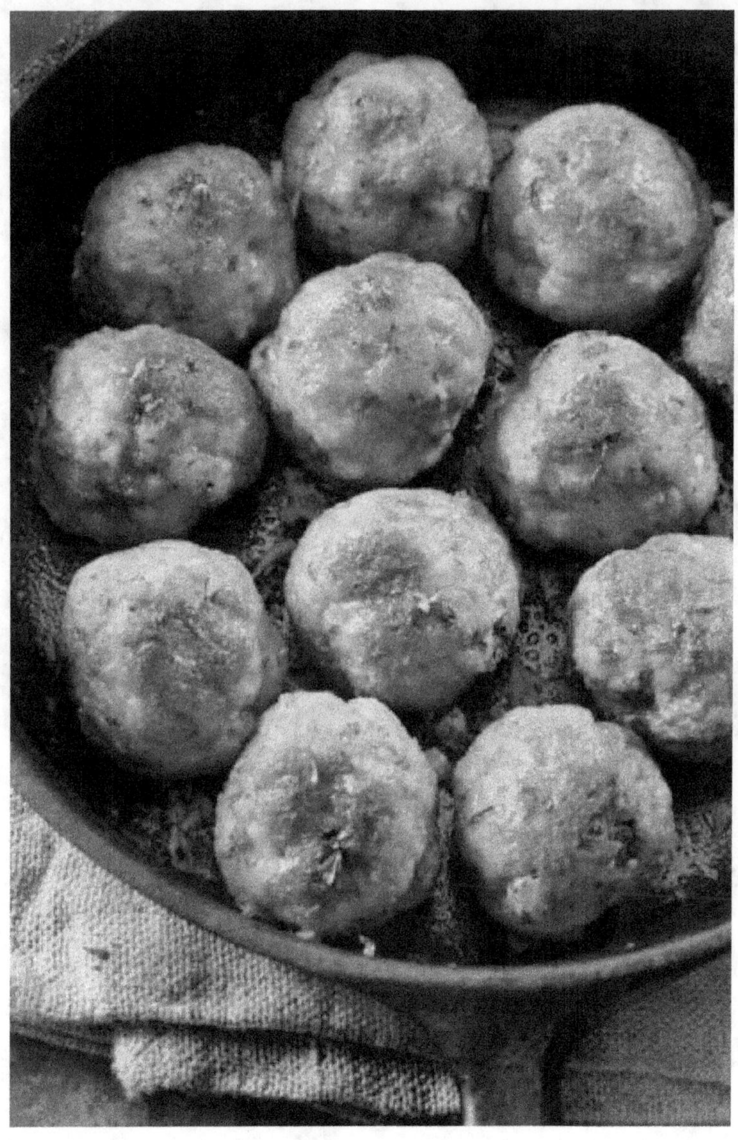

Lemon Herb Grilled Salmon

Preparation Time: 15 minutes
Cooking Time: 10 minutes
Yield: 4 servings

Ingredients:

- 4 salmon fillets
- 2 tablespoons olive oil
- Zest of 1 lemon
- Juice of 1 lemon
- 2 cloves garlic, minced
- 1 teaspoon dried dill
- 1 teaspoon dried thyme
- Salt and black pepper to taste
- Lemon wedges for serving

Procedure:

1. **Preheat Grill:**
   - Preheat the grill to medium-high heat.
2. **Prepare Marinade:**
   - In a bowl, whisk together olive oil, lemon zest, lemon juice, minced garlic, dried dill, dried thyme, salt, and black pepper.
3. **Marinate Salmon:**
   - Place salmon fillets in a shallow dish and coat them with the prepared marinade. Let them marinate for at least 10 minutes.
4. **Grill Salmon:**
   - Grill the salmon fillets for approximately 4-5 minutes per side or until the fish flakes easily with a fork.
5. **Serve:**
   - Serve Lemon Herb Grilled Salmon hot, accompanied by lemon wedges.

Chickpea and Vegetable Stir-Fry

Preparation Time: 20 minutes
Cooking Time: 15 minutes
Yield: 4 servings

Ingredients:

- 2 cups cooked chickpeas
- 1 broccoli crown, cut into florets
- 1 bell pepper, sliced
- 1 carrot, julienned
- 1 zucchini, sliced
- 3 tablespoons soy sauce
- 1 tablespoon hoisin sauce
- 1 tablespoon sesame oil
- 2 cloves garlic, minced
- 1 teaspoon ginger, minced
- Green onions for garnish

Procedure:

1. **Prepare Chickpeas:**
   - If using canned chickpeas, drain and rinse them. If using dried chickpeas, ensure they are cooked and ready.
2. **Stir-Fry Vegetables:**
   - In a wok or large skillet, stir-fry broccoli florets, sliced bell pepper, julienned carrot, and sliced zucchini until they are crisp-tender.
3. **Add Chickpeas:**
   - Add cooked chickpeas to the stir-fried vegetables.
4. **Prepare Sauce:**
   - In a small bowl, whisk together soy sauce, hoisin sauce, sesame oil, minced garlic, and minced ginger.
5. **Combine and Cook:**
   - Pour the sauce over the chickpea and vegetable mixture. Stir well and cook for an additional 2-3 minutes until everything is heated through.
6. **Garnish and Serve:**

- Garnish with chopped green onions and serve Chickpea and Vegetable Stir-Fry over brown rice or quinoa.

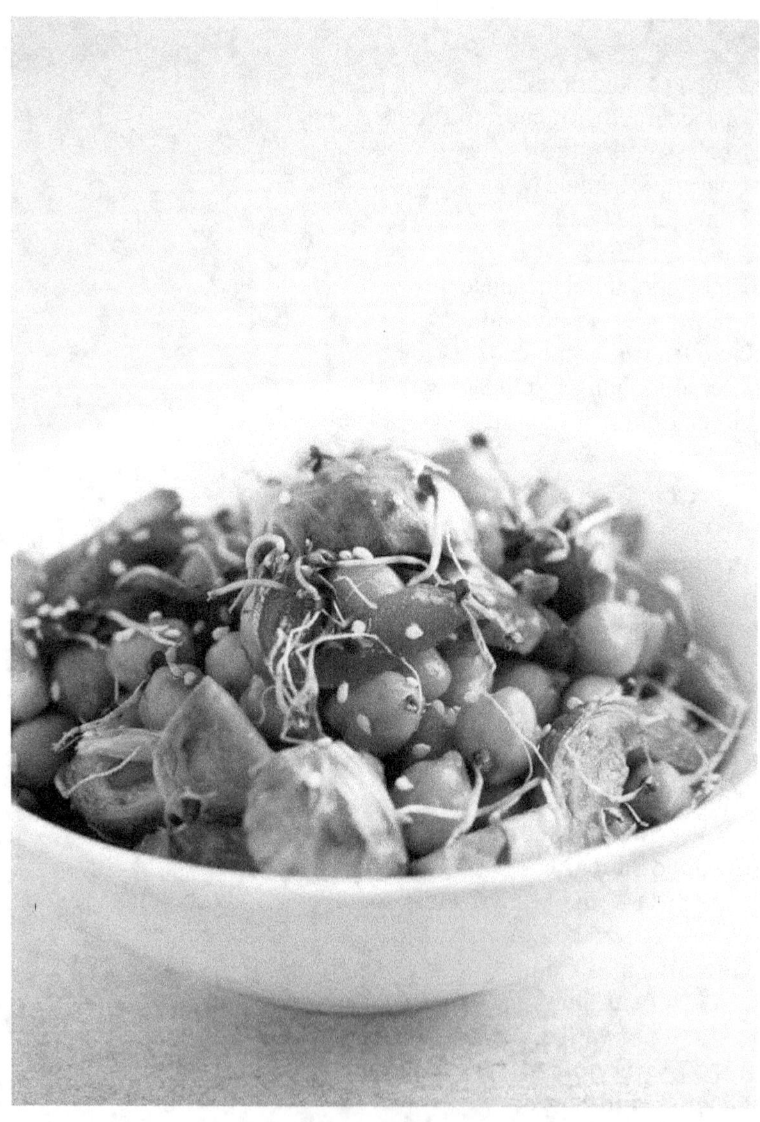

Baked Cod with Lemon and Herbs

Preparation Time: 15 minutes
Cooking Time: 20 minutes
Yield: 4 servings

Ingredients:

- 4 cod fillets
- 3 tablespoons olive oil
- Zest of 1 lemon
- Juice of 1 lemon
- 2 tablespoons fresh parsley, chopped
- 1 teaspoon dried oregano
- 1 teaspoon dried thyme
- Salt and black pepper to taste

Procedure:

1. **Preheat Oven:**
   - Preheat the oven to 400°F (200°C).
2. **Prepare Cod Fillets:**
   - Pat cod fillets dry with paper towels and place them in a baking dish.
3. **Make Herb Mixture:**
   - In a small bowl, combine olive oil, lemon zest, lemon juice, chopped fresh parsley, dried oregano, dried thyme, salt, and black pepper.
4. **Coat and Bake:**
   - Coat the cod fillets with the herb mixture, ensuring even coverage. Bake in the preheated oven for 15-20 minutes or until the fish flakes easily with a fork.
5. **Serve:**
   - Serve Baked Cod with Lemon and Herbs hot, and drizzle with any remaining herb mixture.

Quinoa and Vegetable Stir-Fry

Preparation Time: 20 minutes
Cooking Time: 15 minutes
Yield: 4 servings

Ingredients:

- 1 cup quinoa, rinsed and cooked
- 1 broccoli crown, cut into florets
- 1 red bell pepper, sliced
- 1 yellow bell pepper, sliced
- 1 carrot, julienned
- 3 tablespoons soy sauce
- 1 tablespoon hoisin sauce
- 1 tablespoon sesame oil
- 2 cloves garlic, minced
- 1 teaspoon ginger, minced
- Green onions for garnish

Procedure:

1. **Prepare Quinoa:**
   - Cook quinoa according to package instructions and set aside.
2. **Stir-Fry Vegetables:**
   - In a wok or large skillet, stir-fry broccoli florets, sliced red bell pepper, sliced yellow bell pepper, and julienned carrot until they are crisp-tender.
3. **Add Quinoa:**
   - Add cooked quinoa to the stir-fried vegetables.
4. **Prepare Sauce:**
   - In a small bowl, whisk together soy sauce, hoisin sauce, sesame oil, minced garlic, and minced ginger.
5. **Combine and Cook:**
   - Pour the sauce over the quinoa and vegetable mixture. Stir well and cook for an additional 2-3 minutes until everything is heated through.
6. **Garnish and Serve:**

- Garnish with chopped green onions and serve Quinoa and Vegetable Stir-Fry hot.

Sweet Potato and Chickpea Curry

Preparation Time: 25 minutes
Cooking Time: 25 minutes
Yield: 4 servings

Ingredients:

- 2 large sweet potatoes, peeled and diced
- 1 can (15 oz) chickpeas, drained and rinsed
- 1 onion, finely chopped
- 3 cloves garlic, minced
- 1 can (14 oz) diced tomatoes, undrained
- 1 can (14 oz) coconut milk
- 2 tablespoons curry powder
- 1 teaspoon ground turmeric
- 1 teaspoon ground cumin
- 1 teaspoon paprika
- Salt and black pepper to taste
- Fresh cilantro for garnish

Procedure:

1. **Sauté Onion and Garlic:**
    - In a large pot, sauté finely chopped onion and minced garlic until softened.
2. **Add Spices:**
    - Stir in curry powder, ground turmeric, ground cumin, and paprika. Cook for an additional 2 minutes.
3. **Add Sweet Potatoes and Chickpeas:**
    - Add diced sweet potatoes and drained chickpeas to the pot. Stir to coat them with the spices.
4. **Pour in Tomatoes and Coconut Milk:**

- Pour in undrained diced tomatoes and coconut milk.
  Bring the mixture to a simmer and cook until the sweet
  potatoes are tender.

5. **Adjust Seasoning and Serve:**
   - Season the curry with salt and black pepper to taste.
     Garnish with fresh cilantro and serve Sweet Potato and
     Chickpea Curry hot.

Snacks and sides

Guilt-Free Crunchy Treats

Preparation Time: 10 minutes
Cooking Time: 15 minutes
Yield: 4 servings

Ingredients:

- 2 cups kale, washed and dried
- 1 tablespoon olive oil
- 1/2 teaspoon garlic powder
- 1/2 teaspoon paprika
- Salt to taste

Procedure:

1. **Preheat Oven:**
   - Preheat the oven to 350°F (175°C).
2. **Prepare Kale:**
   - Remove stems from kale leaves and tear them into bite-sized pieces.
3. **Massage with Olive Oil:**
   - In a bowl, massage kale pieces with olive oil until well-coated.
4. **Season and Bake:**
   - Sprinkle garlic powder, paprika, and salt over the kale. Spread the kale on a baking sheet and bake for 10-15 minutes or until crispy.
5. **Cool and Serve:**
   - Allow the kale chips to cool before serving. Enjoy these Guilt-Free Crunchy Treats as a nutritious snack.

Dips and Spreads

Hummus:

Preparation Time: 10 minutes
Yield: 2 cups

Ingredients:
- 1 can (15 oz) chickpeas, drained and rinsed
- 1/4 cup tahini
- 2 cloves garlic, minced
- 2 tablespoons lemon juice
- 2 tablespoons olive oil
- Salt and black pepper to taste

Procedure:
1. **Blend *Ingredients*:**
   - In a food processor, combine chickpeas, tahini, minced garlic, lemon juice, and olive oil. Blend until smooth.
2. **Season and Serve:**
   - Season with salt and black pepper to taste. Transfer to a bowl and serve as a dip.

Salsa:

Preparation Time: 15 minutes
Yield: 2 cups

Ingredients:
- 4 large tomatoes, diced
- 1 onion, finely chopped
- 1 jalapeño, seeded and minced
- 1/4 cup fresh cilantro, chopped
- 2 tablespoons lime juice
- Salt to taste

Procedure:
1. **Combine *Ingredients*:**
     - In a bowl, combine diced tomatoes, finely chopped onion, minced jalapeño, chopped fresh cilantro, and lime juice.
2. **Season and Chill:**
     - Season the salsa with salt to taste. Chill in the refrigerator before serving.
3. **Serve:**
     - Serve the salsa with whole-grain tortilla chips or as a topping for dishes.

Roasted Vegetables

Preparation Time: 15 minutes
Cooking Time: 25 minutes
Yield: 4 servings

Ingredients:

- 2 cups broccoli florets
- 2 cups cauliflower florets
- 1 bell pepper, sliced
- 1 zucchini, sliced
- 2 tablespoons olive oil
- 1 teaspoon dried thyme
- 1 teaspoon garlic powder
- Salt and black pepper to taste

Procedure:

1. **Preheat Oven:**
   - Preheat the oven to 400°F (200°C).
2. **Prepare Vegetables:**
   - In a large bowl, toss broccoli florets, cauliflower florets, sliced bell pepper, and sliced zucchini with olive oil.
3. **Season and Roast:**
   - Sprinkle dried thyme, garlic powder, salt, and black pepper over the vegetables. Spread them on a baking sheet and roast for 20-25 minutes or until golden brown and tender.
4. **Serve:**
   - Serve Roasted Vegetables as a side dish or snack.

Whole Grain Goodness

Preparation Time: 10 minutes
Cooking Time: 20 minutes
Yield: 4 servings

Ingredients:

- 1 cup quinoa, rinsed and cooked
- 1 cup mixed vegetables (peas, carrots, corn)
- 1/4 cup almonds, chopped
- 2 tablespoons fresh parsley, chopped
- 1 tablespoon olive oil
- 1 tablespoon lemon juice
- Salt and black pepper to taste

Procedure:

1. **Prepare Quinoa:**
   - Cook quinoa according to package instructions and set aside.
2. **Sauté Vegetables:**
   - In a skillet, sauté mixed vegetables in olive oil until they are tender.
3. **Combine *Ingredients*:**
   - In a bowl, combine cooked quinoa, sautéed vegetables, chopped almonds, chopped fresh parsley, and lemon juice.
4. **Season and Serve:**
   - Season with salt and black pepper to taste. Serve Whole Grain Goodness as a nutritious side dish.

Mediterranean Cucumber Cups

Preparation Time: 15 minutes
Yield: 4 servings

Ingredients:

- 2 large cucumbers, peeled and sliced into rounds
- 1 cup cherry tomatoes, halved
- 1/2 cup feta cheese, crumbled
- 1/4 cup Kalamata olives, sliced
- 2 tablespoons fresh mint, chopped
- 2 tablespoons balsamic glaze

Procedure:

1. **Prepare Cucumber Cups:**
   - Using a spoon, hollow out the center of each cucumber round to create cups.
2. **Fill with *Ingredients*:**
   - Fill each cucumber cup with cherry tomatoes, crumbled feta cheese, sliced Kalamata olives, and chopped fresh mint.
3. **Drizzle with Balsamic Glaze:**
   - Drizzle balsamic glaze over the Mediterranean Cucumber Cups.
4. **Serve:**
   - Serve as a refreshing and flavorful side or snack.

Hummus-Stuffed Bell Peppers

Preparation Time: 15 minutes
Yield: 4 servings

Ingredients:

- 2 large bell peppers, sliced into halves
- Hummus (store-bought or homemade)
- Cherry tomatoes, halved
- Cucumber, sliced
- Fresh parsley, chopped

Procedure:

1. **Prepare Bell Peppers:**
   - Slice bell peppers into halves and remove seeds.
2. **Fill with Hummus:**
   - Fill each bell pepper half with hummus.
3. **Top with Tomatoes and Cucumber:**
   - Top the hummus-filled peppers with halved cherry tomatoes and sliced cucumber.
4. **Garnish:**
   - Garnish with chopped fresh parsley.
5. **Serve:**
   - Serve Hummus-Stuffed Bell Peppers as a delightful and healthy snack.

Greek Yogurt and Berry Parfait

Preparation Time: 10 minutes
Yield: 2 servings

Ingredients:

- 1 cup Greek yogurt
- Mixed berries (strawberries, blueberries, raspberries)
- Granola
- Honey (optional)

Procedure:

1. **Layer Yogurt:**
   - In a glass or bowl, layer Greek yogurt at the bottom.
2. **Add Berries:**
   - Add a layer of mixed berries over the yogurt.
3. **Sprinkle Granola:**
   - Sprinkle granola on top of the berries.
4. **Repeat Layers:**
   - Repeat the layers until the glass or bowl is filled.
5. **Drizzle with Honey (Optional):**
   - Optionally, drizzle honey over the top for added sweetness.
6. **Serve:**
   - Serve Greek Yogurt and Berry Parfait as a delicious and nutritious snack or dessert.

Caprese Skewers

Preparation Time: 15 minutes
Yield: 4 servings

Ingredients:

- Cherry tomatoes
- Fresh mozzarella balls
- Fresh basil leaves
- Balsamic glaze

Procedure:

1. **Assemble Skewers:**
   - Thread a cherry tomato, a fresh mozzarella ball, and a fresh basil leaf onto small skewers.
2. **Arrange on Platter:**
   - Arrange the Caprese skewers on a serving platter.
3. **Drizzle with Balsamic Glaze:**
   - Drizzle balsamic glaze over the assembled skewers.
4. **Serve:**
   - Serve Caprese Skewers as a delightful and elegant snack

Cucumber and Carrot Sticks with Tzatziki

Preparation Time: 10 minutes
Yield: 4 servings

Ingredients:

- Cucumber, cut into sticks
- Carrots, cut into sticks
- Tzatziki sauce (store-bought or homemade)

Procedure:

1. **Prepare Vegetables:**
   - Cut cucumber and carrots into sticks.
2. **Serve with Tzatziki:**
   - Arrange the cucumber and carrot sticks on a plate and serve with tzatziki sauce for dipping.
3. **Enjoy:**
   - Enjoy Cucumber and Carrot Sticks with Tzatziki as a refreshing and crunchy snack.

Quinoa and Black Bean Salad

Preparation Time: 20 minutes
Yield: 4 servings

Ingredients:

- 1 cup quinoa, rinsed and cooked
- 1 can (15 oz) black beans, drained and rinsed
- Cherry tomatoes, halved
- Red onion, finely chopped
- Fresh cilantro, chopped
- Lime juice
- Olive oil
- Salt and black pepper to taste

Procedure:

1. **Combine *Ingredients*:**
   - In a bowl, combine cooked quinoa, black beans, cherry tomatoes, finely chopped red onion, and chopped fresh cilantro.
2. **Make Dressing:**
   - In a small bowl, whisk together lime juice, olive oil, salt, and black pepper.
3. **Toss and Chill:**
   - Pour the dressing over the quinoa mixture and toss until well combined. Chill in the refrigerator for at least 15 minutes.
4. **Serve:**
   - Serve Quinoa and Black Bean Salad as a flavorful and satisfying side dish or snack.

Spinach and Artichoke Dip

Preparation Time: 15 minutes
Cooking Time: 20 minutes
Yield: 4 servings

Ingredients:

- 2 cups fresh spinach, chopped
- 1 can (14 oz) artichoke hearts, drained and chopped
- 1 cup Greek yogurt
- 1/2 cup mayonnaise
- 1 cup Parmesan cheese, grated
- 1 cup mozzarella cheese, shredded
- 2 cloves garlic, minced
- Salt and black pepper to taste
- Whole-grain pita chips for serving

Procedure:

1. **Preheat Oven:**
   - Preheat the oven to 375°F (190°C).
2. **Prepare Spinach and Artichokes:**
   - In a bowl, combine chopped spinach and chopped artichoke hearts.
3. **Make Dip Mixture:**
   - In another bowl, mix Greek yogurt, mayonnaise, Parmesan cheese, mozzarella cheese, minced garlic, salt, and black pepper.
4. **Combine and Bake:**
   - Combine the spinach and artichoke mixture with the dip mixture. Transfer to a baking dish and bake for 20 minutes or until bubbly and golden.
5. **Serve:**
   - Serve Spinach and Artichoke Dip with whole-grain pita chips for a tasty and satisfying snack.

Avocado and Tomato Salsa

Preparation Time: 10 minutes
Yield: 2 cups

Ingredients:

- 2 avocados, diced
- 1 cup cherry tomatoes, diced
- Red onion, finely chopped
- Fresh cilantro, chopped
- Lime juice
- Salt and black pepper to taste
- Whole-grain tortilla chips for serving

Procedure:

1. **Combine *Ingredients*:**
   - In a bowl, combine diced avocados, diced cherry tomatoes, finely chopped red onion, and chopped fresh cilantro.
2. **Add Lime Juice:**
   - Drizzle lime juice over the mixture.
3. **Season:**
   - Season with salt and black pepper to taste.
4. **Mix and Serve:**
   - Gently mix the *ingredients* and serve Avocado and Tomato Salsa with whole-grain tortilla chips for a delightful snack.

Roasted Red Pepper Hummus

Preparation Time: 10 minutes
Yield: 2 cups

Ingredients:

- 1 can (15 oz) chickpeas, drained and rinsed
- 1/2 cup roasted red peppers, drained
- 1/4 cup tahini
- 2 cloves garlic, minced
- Lemon juice
- Olive oil
- Paprika for garnish
- Baby carrots and cucumber slices for dipping

Procedure:

1. **Blend *Ingredients*:**
   - In a food processor, blend chickpeas, roasted red peppers, tahini, minced garlic, and a splash of lemon juice.
2. **Stream in Olive Oil:**
   - While the food processor is running, stream in olive oil until the hummus reaches a smooth consistency.
3. **Adjust Seasoning:**
   - Adjust the flavor with additional lemon juice or salt if needed.
4. **Garnish and Serve:**
   - Transfer the hummus to a bowl, drizzle with olive oil, sprinkle with paprika, and serve with baby carrots and cucumber slices.

Quinoa-Stuffed Mushrooms

Preparation Time: 20 minutes
Cooking Time: 25 minutes
Yield: 4 servings

Ingredients:

- 8 large mushrooms, stems removed
- 1 cup quinoa, cooked
- Spinach, chopped
- Feta cheese, crumbled
- Cherry tomatoes, diced
- Olive oil
- Garlic powder
- Salt and black pepper to taste

Procedure:

1. **Preheat Oven:**
   - Preheat the oven to 375°F (190°C).
2. **Prepare Mushrooms:**
   - Clean mushrooms and remove stems.
3. **Sauté Spinach:**
   - In a skillet, sauté chopped spinach in olive oil until wilted.
4. **Mix Quinoa Filling:**
   - In a bowl, mix cooked quinoa, sautéed spinach, crumbled feta cheese, diced cherry tomatoes, garlic powder, salt, and black pepper.
5. **Stuff Mushrooms:**
   - Stuff each mushroom cap with the quinoa filling.
6. **Bake:**
   - Place stuffed mushrooms on a baking sheet and bake for 20-25 minutes or until mushrooms are tender.
7. **Serve:**
   - Serve Quinoa-Stuffed Mushrooms as a savory and wholesome snack.

Greek Salad Skewers

Preparation Time: 15 minutes
Yield: 4 servings

Ingredients:

- Cherry tomatoes
- Cucumber, cut into chunks
- Feta cheese, cubed
- Kalamata olives
- Red onion, sliced
- Greek salad dressing

Procedure:

1. **Assemble Skewers:**
   - Thread cherry tomatoes, cucumber chunks, feta cheese cubes, Kalamata olives, and slices of red onion onto small skewers.
2. **Drizzle with Dressing:**
   - Drizzle Greek salad dressing over the assembled skewers.
3. **Serve:**
   - Serve Greek Salad Skewers as a refreshing and flavorful side or snack.

Quinoa and Vegetable Spring Rolls

Preparation Time: 20 minutes
Yield: 8 spring rolls

Ingredients:

- Rice paper wrappers
- 1 cup quinoa, cooked
- Carrots, julienned
- Cucumber, julienned
- Bell peppers, thinly sliced
- Fresh cilantro leaves
- Mint leaves
- Soy sauce or tamari for dipping

Procedure:

1. **Prepare Rice Paper Wrappers:**
   - Dip rice paper wrappers in warm water until softened.
2. **Assemble Spring Rolls:**
   - On each wrapper, place a portion of cooked quinoa, julienned carrots, cucumber, sliced bell peppers, cilantro leaves, and mint leaves.
3. **Roll and Seal:**
   - Roll the wrappers, folding in the sides, to form spring rolls. Seal the edges.
4. **Slice and Serve:**
   - Slice the spring rolls diagonally and serve with soy sauce or tamari for dipping.
5. **Enjoy:**
   - Enjoy Quinoa and Vegetable Spring Rolls as a light and satisfying snack.

Baked Sweet Potato Fries

Preparation Time: 15 minutes
Cooking Time: 25 minutes
Yield: 4 servings

Ingredients:

- 2 large sweet potatoes, cut into fries
- Olive oil
- Paprika
- Garlic powder
- Salt and black pepper to taste

Procedure:

1. **Preheat Oven***:*
   - Preheat the oven to 425°F (220°C).
2. **Coat Sweet Potatoes:**
   - In a bowl, toss sweet potato fries with olive oil, paprika, garlic powder, salt, and black pepper.
3. **Spread on Baking Sheet:**
   - Spread the seasoned sweet potato fries on a baking sheet in a single layer.
4. **Bake:**
   - Bake for 20-25 minutes, turning halfway through, until the fries are golden and crisp.
5. **Serve:**
   - Serve Baked Sweet Potato Fries as a flavorful and nutritious side or snack.

Mediterranean Chickpea Salad

Preparation Time: 15 minutes
Yield: 4 servings

Ingredients:

- 2 cans (15 oz each) chickpeas, drained and rinsed
- Cherry tomatoes, halved
- Cucumber, diced
- Red onion, finely chopped
- Kalamata olives, sliced
- Feta cheese, crumbled
- Fresh parsley, chopped
- Olive oil
- Red wine vinegar
- Dried oregano
- Salt and black pepper to taste

Procedure:

1. **Combine *Ingredients*:**
   - In a large bowl, combine chickpeas, cherry tomatoes, diced cucumber, finely chopped red onion, sliced Kalamata olives, crumbled feta cheese, and chopped fresh parsley.
2. **Make Dressing:**
   - In a small bowl, whisk together olive oil, red wine vinegar, dried oregano, salt, and black pepper.
3. **Toss and Serve:**
   - Pour the dressing over the salad and toss until well combined. Serve Mediterranean Chickpea Salad as a refreshing and protein-packed side.

Desserts for Dash Enthusiasts

Fruity Delights

Fruit Salad with Honey-Lime Drizzle:

Preparation Time: 15 minutes
Yield: 4 servings

Ingredients:

- Assorted fresh fruits (strawberries, blueberries, pineapple, kiwi, etc.)
- Fresh mint leaves for garnish
- Honey
- Lime juice

Procedure:

1. **Prepare Fruits:**
   - Wash, peel, and chop the assorted fresh fruits into bite-sized pieces.
2. **Create Fruit Salad:**
   - In a bowl, combine the assorted fruits.
3. **Prepare Honey-Lime Drizzle:**
   - In a small bowl, mix honey and lime juice to create the drizzle.
4. **Drizzle and Toss:**
   - Drizzle the honey-lime mixture over the fruit salad and toss gently to coat.
5. **Garnish and Serve:**
   - Garnish with fresh mint leaves and serve this refreshing Fruit Salad with Honey-Lime Drizzle as a delightful dessert.

Healthy Baking Secrets

Baked Apples with Cinnamon and Almonds:

Preparation Time: 15 minutes
Cooking Time: 30 minutes
Yield: 4 servings

Ingredients:

- 4 apples, cored and halved
- Cinnamon
- Almonds, chopped
- Honey (optional)

Procedure:

1. **Preheat Oven:**
   - Preheat the oven to 375°F (190°C).
2. **Prepare Apples:**
   - Core and halve the apples.
3. **Sprinkle with Cinnamon:**
   - Sprinkle the apple halves with cinnamon.
   Add Chopped Almonds:

   - Sprinkle chopped almonds over the apples.
4. **Bake:**
   - Place the apples on a baking sheet and bake for 25-30 minutes or until tender.
5. **Optional Drizzle:**
   - Drizzle with honey if desired before serving these Baked Apples with Cinnamon and Almonds.

Indulgent Treats in Moderation
Dark Chocolate-Dipped Strawberries:

Preparation Time: 15 minutes
Yield: 12 strawberries

Ingredients:

- Fresh strawberries, washed and dried
- Dark chocolate, melted
- Chopped nuts or shredded coconut (optional)

Procedure:

1. **Melt Chocolate:**
   - Melt dark chocolate in a heatproof bowl.
2. **Dip Strawberries:**
   - Dip each strawberry into the melted chocolate, covering it partially.
3. **Optional Toppings:**
   - If desired, sprinkle chopped nuts or shredded coconut over the chocolate.
4. **Place on Tray:**
   - Place the chocolate-dipped strawberries on a tray lined with parchment paper.
5. **Chill and Serve:**
   - Chill in the refrigerator until the chocolate sets. Serve these Dark Chocolate-Dipped Strawberries as a sweet and guilt-free indulgence.

Sweet Potato and Banana Bites

Preparation Time: 20 minutes
Cooking Time: 20 minutes
Yield: 12 bites

Ingredients:

- 1 sweet potato, peeled and grated
- 1 ripe banana, mashed
- Cinnamon
- Nutmeg
- Chopped walnuts (optional)

Procedure:

1. **Preheat Oven:**
   - Preheat the oven to 375°F (190°C).
2. **Combine *Ingredients*:**
   - In a bowl, combine grated sweet potato, mashed banana, cinnamon, nutmeg, and chopped walnuts if using.
3. **Form Bites:**
   - Form the mixture into bite-sized rounds and place them on a baking sheet.
4. **Bake:**
   - Bake for 20 minutes or until the edges are golden.
5. **Cool and Enjoy:**
   - Allow the Sweet Potato and Banana Bites to cool before serving.

Berry and Yogurt Parfait

Preparation Time: 10 minutes
Yield: 4 servings

Ingredients:

- Mixed berries (strawberries, blueberries, raspberries)
- Greek yogurt
- Granola
- Honey (optional)

Procedure:

1. **Layer Yogurt:**
   - In glasses or bowls, layer Greek yogurt at the bottom.
2. **Add Berries:**
   - Add a layer of mixed berries over the yogurt.
3. **Sprinkle Granola:**
   - Sprinkle granola on top of the berries.
4. **Repeat Layers:**
   - Repeat the layers until the glass or bowl is filled.
5. **Drizzle with Honey (Optional):**
   - Optionally, drizzle honey over the top for added sweetness.
6. **Serve:**
   - Serve Berry and Yogurt Parfait as a delicious and wholesome dessert.

Berry and Almond Frozen Yogurt Bites

Preparation Time: 15 minutes
Freezing Time: 2 hours
Yield: 12 bites

Ingredients:

- Greek yogurt
- Mixed berries (strawberries, blueberries, raspberries)
- Almonds, chopped
- Honey (optional)

Procedure:

1. **Prepare Yogurt Mixture:**
   - In a bowl, mix Greek yogurt with chopped almonds and honey if desired.
2. **Add Berries:**
   - Gently fold in mixed berries into the yogurt mixture.
3. **Spoon into Molds:**
   - Spoon the yogurt mixture into silicone molds or ice cube trays.
4. **Freeze:**
   - Freeze for at least 2 hours or until firm.

Chia Seed Pudding with Mango

Preparation Time: 10 minutes
Chilling Time: 4 hours or overnight
Yield: 4 servings

Ingredients:

- Chia seeds
- Almond milk (or any preferred milk)
- Mango, diced
- Vanilla extract
- Maple syrup (optional)

Procedure:

1. **Mix Chia Pudding:**
   - In a bowl, mix chia seeds, almond milk, vanilla extract, and maple syrup if desired. Stir well.
2. **Add Mango:**
   - Gently fold in diced mango into the chia seed mixture.
3. **Chill:**
   - Refrigerate for at least 4 hours or overnight to allow the chia seeds to absorb the liquid.
4. **Stir and Serve:**
   - Before serving, stir the pudding and top with additional mango if desired. Serve this Chia Seed Pudding with Mango as a delightful and nutritious dessert.

Banana and Walnut Oat Cookies

Preparation Time: 15 minutes
Baking Time: 12-15 minutes
Yield: 12 cookies

Ingredients:

- Rolled oats
- Ripe bananas, mashed
- Walnuts, chopped
- Cinnamon
- Vanilla extract

Procedure:

1. **Preheat Oven:**
   - Preheat the oven to 350°F (180°C).
2. **Mix *Ingredients*:**
   - In a bowl, mix rolled oats, mashed bananas, chopped walnuts, cinnamon, and vanilla extract.
3. **Shape Cookies:**
   - Drop spoonfuls of the mixture onto a baking sheet, shaping them into cookies.
4. **Bake:**
   - Bake for 12-15 minutes or until the edges are golden.
5. **Cool and Enjoy:**
   - Allow the Banana and Walnut Oat Cookies to cool before serving.

Dark Chocolate and Raspberry Parfait

Preparation Time: 15 minutes
Yield: 4 servings

Ingredients:

- Dark chocolate, melted
- Greek yogurt
- Fresh raspberries
- Almond slices

Procedure:

1. **Layer Greek Yogurt:**
   - In glasses or bowls, layer Greek yogurt at the bottom.
2. **Drizzle with Chocolate:**
   - Drizzle melted dark chocolate over the yogurt layer.
3. **Add Raspberries:**
   - Add a layer of fresh raspberries.
4. **Repeat Layers:**
   - Repeat the layers until the glass or bowl is filled.
5. **Top with Almonds:**
   - Top the parfait with almond slices.
6. **Serve:**
   - Serve Dark Chocolate and Raspberry Parfait as a decadent and satisfying dessert.

Mango and Coconut Chia Popsicles

Preparation Time: 10 minutes
Freezing Time: 4 hours or overnight
Yield: 6 popsicles

Ingredients:

- Mango, diced
- Coconut milk
- Chia seeds

Procedure:

1. **Blend Mango:**
   - Blend diced mango until smooth.
2. **Mix Chia Mixture:**
   - In a bowl, mix coconut milk and chia seeds. Let it sit for a few minutes until it thickens.
3. **Layer in Popsicle Molds:**
   - Alternate layers of mango puree and chia mixture in popsicle molds.
4. **Insert Sticks:**
   - Insert popsicle sticks and freeze for at least 4 hours or overnight.
5. **Unmold and Enjoy:**
   - Unmold the Mango and Coconut Chia Popsicles and enjoy this tropical and healthy frozen treat.

Special Occasion Menus

Hosting Dash-Friendly Gatherings: Entertaining guests while staying true to the Dash Diet principles can be both enjoyable and health-conscious. Create a welcoming atmosphere with dishes that align with the Dash Diet. Your guests will savor the flavors of nutritious and delicious options suitable for any gathering.

Appetizer Extravaganza: Kick off your gathering with a selection of mouthwatering appetizers. Opt for fresh vegetable platters featuring vibrant colors and diverse textures. Pair them with yogurt-based dips infused with herbs for a delightful burst of flavor. Whole-grain crackers complemented by lean protein choices like smoked salmon or hummus ensure a sophisticated start to your event.

Main Course Marvels: Crafting a main course menu that emphasizes lean proteins, abundant vegetables, and whole grains is key. Consider grilled chicken skewers with a zesty citrus marinade or quinoa-stuffed bell peppers for a plant-based option. Balanced and hearty, these dishes ensure a satisfying and heart-healthy meal for your guests.

Dessert Delights: Indulge in sweet treats without compromising on health. Consider desserts that incorporate fresh fruits, such as a berry parfait with Greek yogurt or a dark chocolate-dipped fruit platter. For a creative touch, offer a selection of fruit-based sorbets or yogurt-based frozen treats. These options provide a guilt-free conclusion to your gathering.

Holiday Feasts: Maintaining the Dash Diet during holidays doesn't mean sacrificing flavor and tradition. Prepare festive feasts that celebrate the season while adhering to Dash Diet principles. From Thanksgiving to Christmas, ensure your holiday table is filled with dishes that prioritize health without compromising on taste.

Turkey Day Triumphs: Rethink classic Thanksgiving dishes with a Dash Diet twist. Consider a herb-infused roasted turkey as the centerpiece, complemented by cranberry-orange quinoa stuffing. Sides like roasted Brussels sprouts and sweet potato casserole with a pecan crust add both nutrition and flavor to your holiday feast.

Christmas Classics, Dash-Style: Create a Christmas spread that balances festive flavors with heart-healthy choices. Opt for dishes like herb-roasted lamb or a baked salmon fillet with a citrus glaze. Accompany these main courses with sides such as quinoa salad with pomegranate and roasted root vegetables, ensuring your holiday dinner is a celebration of health and happiness.

Celebratory Events

Whether it's birthdays, anniversaries, or other special milestones, you can celebrate in style while adhering to the Dash Diet. Discover innovative ways to mark special occasions with menus that prioritize well-being, ensuring that joyous events are also heart-healthy.

Birthday Bashes with a Dash: Plan birthday celebrations with delicious and nutritious alternatives. Consider serving a fruit-infused birthday cake or a yogurt-based parfait station with various toppings. Incorporate colorful and flavorful dishes like grilled shrimp skewers and vegetable kebabs to create a festive atmosphere.

Anniversary Elegance: Celebrate years of love and commitment with a romantic and heart-healthy anniversary dinner. Begin with a seafood appetizer like shrimp cocktail or oysters, followed by a main course featuring grilled fish or lean cuts of beef. Conclude the meal with a sophisticated fruit and dark chocolate fondue for a touch of indulgence.

Dash Diet and Beyond

Lifestyle Tips for Long-Term Success

Achieving long-term success with the Dash Diet involves adopting a sustainable lifestyle. Uncover practical tips and habits that will support your health journey, making Dash Diet principles an integral part of your daily life.

Meal Planning Mastery: Effective meal planning is a cornerstone of Dash Diet success. Learn how to plan and organize meals in advance, ensuring a week of nutritious and balanced eating. Explore batch cooking techniques to save time and make healthy choices effortlessly.

Smart Grocery Shopping: Navigate the grocery store with ease, making informed choices that align with the Dash Diet. Understand how to read food labels, choose fresh produce, and identify whole grains. Empower yourself to shop for health and maintain a well-stocked kitchen.

Staying Active and Fit

A healthy lifestyle extends beyond the kitchen. Explore ways to stay active and fit, complementing your dietary choices with physical well-being practices that support overall health.

Fitness for All Ages: Tailor fitness routines to different age groups, ensuring that everyone in the family can participate in activities that promote cardiovascular health and strength. From family walks to group fitness classes, find enjoyable ways to stay active together.

Incorporating Exercise into Daily Life: Discover simple yet effective ways to incorporate exercise into your daily routine. Whether it's taking brisk walks during breaks or incorporating home workouts into your schedule, find the right balance for your lifestyle. Embrace physical activity as a joyful and integral part of your day.

Mindful Eating Practices

Cultivate mindful eating habits that enhance your relationship with food. Learn to savor each bite, recognize hunger and fullness cues, and appreciate the nourishment that comes from Dash Diet-friendly choices.

The Art of Mindful Dining: Embrace the concept of mindful dining, focusing on the sensory experience of each meal. From savoring flavors to being present at the table, discover how mindfulness can enhance your eating habits. Create a calm and enjoyable atmosphere during meals, promoting a positive relationship with food.

Listening to Your Body: Tune in to your body's signals and foster a healthy relationship with food. Understand hunger and fullness cues, making informed choices that align with your body's needs. Develop an awareness of how different foods make you feel and cultivate an intuitive approach to eating.

Appendix

Dash Diet Measurement Conversions

A handy reference for converting measurements, ensuring accuracy and consistency in your Dash Diet cooking and meal preparation. Easily convert between metric and imperial units to follow recipes seamlessly.

Recommended Reading and Resources

Explore additional reading materials and resources that delve deeper into the Dash Diet, providing valuable insights and guidance for your health journey. Discover books, websites, and tools that can support your understanding and implementation of the Dash Diet.

Index

A comprehensive index for quick reference, allowing you to navigate through the cookbook with ease and find the information you need promptly. Easily locate recipes, tips, and specific topics to enhance your Dash Diet experience.

Meal Planner

www.ingramcontent.com/pod-product-compliance
Lightning Source LLC
Chambersburg PA
CBHW070939260726
48661CB00003B/1037